The Complete Keto Dinner Recipe Book

An Amazing Collection of Keto Recipes to Boost Your Dinner and Improve Your Skills

I0145928

Gerard Short

Table of Contents

Caesar Salad

Prep time: 15 minutes | Cook time: 20 minutes | Serves 4

Marcos: Fat 78% | Protein 20% | Carbs 2%

Iowe my uncle a lot since he was the one that introduced me to Caesar salad. As a kid I always thought that salads were never meant to be tasty; however, I could recall the first time I tasted Caesar salad and the way I enjoyed it. The rich, and wonderful taste of the anchovy. The crustiness on each bite that makes it so exquisite. Enjoy this easy to make meal.

You could add edible flowers or even croutons, but they are totally optional

¾ pound (340 g) chicken breasts

1 tablespoon olive oil

Salt and freshly ground black pepper, to taste

3 ounces (85 g) bacon

7 ounces (198 g) Romaine lettuce

1 ounce (28 g) of freshly grate d Parmesan cheese

DRESSING:

½ cup mayonnaise, keto-friendly

1 tablespoon Dijon mustard

½ lemon, juice and zest

½ ounce (14 g) grated Parmesan cheese, finely grated

2 tablespoons anchovy paste

1 garlic clove, finely chopped or pressed

Salt and freshly ground black pepper, to taste

1. Preheat the oven to 350°F (180°C).

2. Spread the chicken breasts in a greased baking dish.

3. Add salt and pepper to the chicken, then drizzle melted butter or olive oil on top of it.

4. Bake the chicken in the preheated oven for 20 minutes, or until you notice that it's fully cooked through by sticking a knife into the thickest part, and making sure that the juices are colorless and smooth. (You can also check by using a cooking thermometer in the thick part, its fully cooked when it reaches 180°F (82°C)). you could also cook the chicken by using the stovetop.

5. Fry the bacon until it gets crispy. Chop the lettuce and put it as a base on two plates, then place the crispy, crumbles bacon on top of the sliced pieces of chicken.

6. In order to make the dressing, put the ingredients in a bowl and mix them with a whisk or with an immersion blender, then set it aside in the refrigerator.

7. End it with a good dollop of dressing and a fine grating of the cheese.

STORAGE: It lasts for about 3 to 5 days in the refrigerator, but it might lose the crispiness on the second day.

REHEAT: You could heat the cold left-over sliced chicken pieces by frying them in a small amount of butter for a delicious, warm addition.

SERVE IT WITH: If you want to serve it side by side with something, then you can make the salad basically go with any type of meat of your choice.

PER SERVING

calories: 521 | fat: 44.5g | total carbs: 4.4g | fiber: 1.3g | protein: 26.0g

Chicken Provençale
Marcos: Fat 77% | Protein 20% | Carbs 3%

Prep time: 10 minutes | Cook time: 45 minutes | Serves 6 to 8

Do you want to have a quick trip to France in the middle of a busy week? Then you must try this chicken Provençale. I tried it the first time when I travelled to France for a week with my family, and ever since then, this meal has a special place in my heart for its unique flavor that I don't get to taste in everyday meals. The perfect balance between the ingredients in this dish takes it to a whole different level from every day to day meals, so treat yourself with an exquisite meal.

2 pounds (907 g) chicken drumsticks

8 ounces (227 g) tomatoes

2½ ounces (71 g) pitted black olives

¼ cup olive oil

5 sliced garlic cloves

1 tablespoon dried oregano

Salt and freshly ground black pepper, to taste

FOR SERVING:

7 ounces (198 g) lettuce

1 cup mayonnaise, keto-friendly

¼ lemon zest

1 tablespoon paprika powder

Salt and freshly ground black pepper, to taste

1. Start by preheating the oven to 400°F (205°C). Set the chicken's skin side up in an oven-safe baking dish. Add olives, garlic and tomatoes on top of the meat and around it.
2. Drizzle over it a good amount of olive oil, then spatter it with oregano and put salt and pepper to season.
3. Put in the oven and roast. It should take about 45 to 60 minutes, depending on the size of the pieces. You can check internal temperature with a meat thermometer. When the temperature reaches 180°F (82°C), the chicken is cooked through. However, you could check by sticking a knife into the thickest part of the chicken, and making sure that the juices run clear.
4. Serve it with a salad of your choice, mayo, lemon zest, and paprika or a mild chili and a sprinkle of salt and pepper.

STORAGE: It could last for up to 4 days in a refrigerator. Allow it to cool first then wrap very well, and make sure it's away from any raw meat. It stays in the freezer for a good 2 months.

REHEAT: It could be reheated in the oven at 350ºF (180ºC) for about 20 minutes, and make sure you keep stirring occasionally, or by using the microwave for about 5 minutes at medium-high.

SERVE IT WITH: It could be served with salads such as the classic Greek salad or any type of keto salads of your choice.

PER SERVING calories: 606 | fat: 51.8g | total carbs: 5.7g | fiber: 2.1g | protein: 29.0g

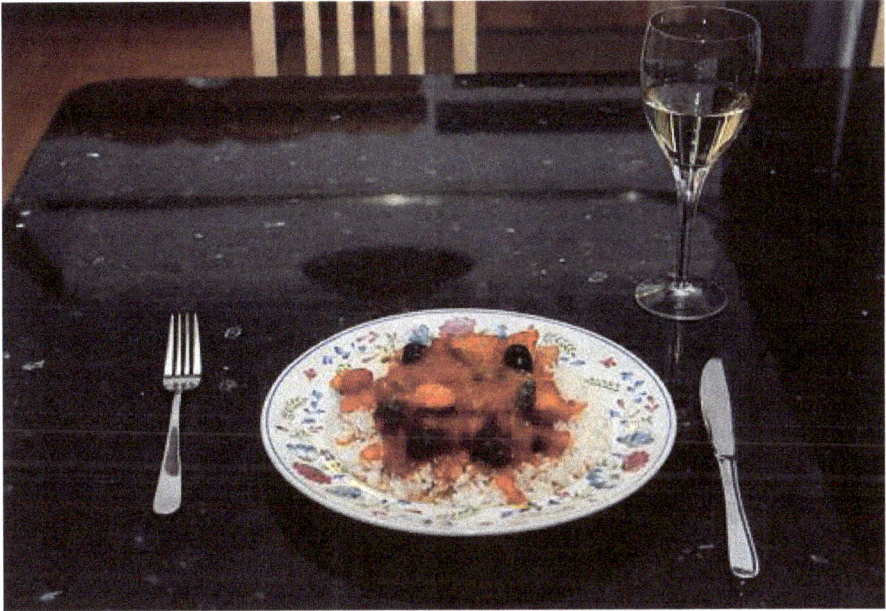

Chicken Breast Wrapped with Bacon And Cauliflower Purée

Macros: Fat 73% | Protein 22% | Carbs 5%

Prep time: 10 minutes | Cook time: 30 minutes | Serves 4

Have you ever thought of a meal so fancy yet so easy to make? Well, you've arrived to your destination. This bacon-wrapped chicken breast is one of my favorite meals to make, everything about it is convenient. It pretty much takes no effort to make, and exquisite at the same time. I grew up in a household full of different people with different tastes, yet they almost never refused to eat the mouth-watering bacon-wrapped chicken.

CAULIFLOWER PURÉE:

4 garlic cloves

2 ounces (57 g) butter

¾ pound (340 g) cauliflower

⅓ cup heavy whipping cream

Salt and freshly ground black pepper, to taste

CHICKEN BREAST:

1 pound (454 g) chicken breast

10 ounces (284 g) bacon

2 tablespoons olive oil

Salt and freshly ground black pepper, to taste

1 pound (454 g) fresh spinach

1. Slightly mash the garlic cloves by pressing hard on them with the handle of a knife, then peel the skin off. Fry them with butter over medium heat until they turn golden. Be careful because it can go from golden to burned in a blink of an eye, and you certainly don't want a bitter taste in your food. Turn off the heat and keep the garlic in the pan while you do the rest.

2. Rinse then trim the cauliflower and divide to smaller florets. Start cooking them in lightly salted water until they are tender, then remove the florets with a strainer and keep some of the water.

3. Place the cauliflower in a food processor or in a blender. Add garlic cloves and the pan juices. The pan juices will add tasty flavor!

4. Add the cream and the purée until it turns smooth. If you wanted it thinner you could add a little bit of the reserved water to the purée. Begin with a couple of tablespoons of reserved water and keep adding more if needed, until it becomes as you desired. Season with salt and pepper to taste.

5. Wrap each chicken breast with one or two pieces of bacon. Put them gently in a pan and fry with olive oil until the bacon is crisp and chicken is cooked through. Keep the pan over low temperature or you could cook them in a hot oven (400°F / 205°C) for 15 minutes until an instant read thermometer inserted in the center of the chicken registers at least 165°F (74°C).

6. Take the chicken off the pan and keep it warm. Use the same pan to fry the spinach, then Serve im mediately with the purée.

STORAGE: The purée could be prepared ahead and stored in the refrigerator for 3 days. However, It lasts up to a month in the freezer, but be sure to keep it in a freezer-safe container.

REHEAT: In order to reheat it you can place it on a dry skillet over medium heat until it gets warm enough.

SERVE IT WITH: You can serve it with salads such as Keto Broccoli salad, or Parmesan Brussels Sprouts Salad.

PER SERVING

calories: 700 | fat: 57.3g | total carbs: 10.3g | fiber: 4.3g | protein: 38.3g

Veggie Beef Stew with Root Mash
<u>Ingredients</u> for 2 servings

½ lb stewing beef, cut into chunks

½ cauliflower head, cut into florets

1 tbsp olive oil

1 parsnip, chopped

1 garlic clove, minced

1 onion, chopped

1 celery stalk, chopped

Salt and black pepper to taste

1 ¼ cups beef stock

2 bay leaves

1 carrot, chopped

½ tbsp rosemary, chopped

1 tomato, chopped

2 tbsp red wine

½ celeriac, chopped

2 tbsp butter

<u>Directions</u> and Total Time: approx. 2 hours 10 minutes

In a pot, cook the celery, onion, and garlic in warm oil over medium heat for 5 minutes. Stir in the beef chunks, and cook for 3 minutes. Season with salt and black pepper. Deglaze the bottom of the pot by adding the red wine. Add in the carrot, parsnip, beef stock, tomato, and bay leaves. Boil the mixture, reduce the heat to low, and cook for 1 hour and 30 minutes.

Meanwhile, heat a pot with water over medium heat. Place in the celeriac, cover, and simmer for 10 minutes. Add in the cauliflower florets, cook for 15 minutes, drain everything, and combine with butter, pepper, and salt. Mash using a potato masher and split the mash between 2 plates. Top with vegetable mixture and stewed beef, sprinkle with rosemary, and serve.

Per serving: Cal 465; Fat 24g; Net Carbs 9.8g; Protein 3.2g

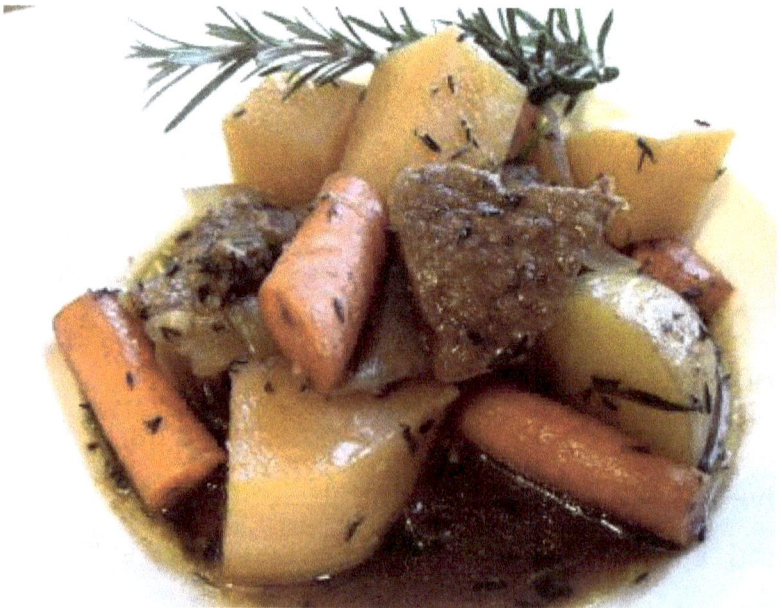

King Size Burgers

Ingredients for 4 servings

2 tbsp olive oil

1 lb ground beef

2 green onions, chopped

1 garlic clove, minced

1 tbsp thyme

2 tbsp almond flour

2 tbsp cup beef broth

½ tbsp chopped parsley

½ tbsp Worcestershire sauce

Directions and Total Time: approx. 25 minutes

Preheat a grill to 370 F Combine all ingredients except for the parsley in a bowl. Mix well with your hands and make 2 patties out of the mixture. Arrange on a lined baking sheet. Bake for about 18-20 minutes, until nice and crispy. Serve sprinkled with parsley.

Per serving: Cal 363; Fat 26g; Net Carbs 3.1g; Protein 25g

Portobello Beef Cheeseburgers

Ingredients for 2 servings

2 tbsp olive oil

½ lb ground beef

½ tsp fresh parsley, chopped

½ tsp Worcestershire sauce

Salt and black pepper to taste

2 slices mozzarella cheese

2 portobello mushroom caps

Directions and Total Time: approx. 25 minutes

In a bowl, mix the beef, parsley, Worcestershire sauce, salt, and black pepper with your hands until evenly combined. Make medium-sized patties out of the mixture.

Preheat a grill to 400 F and coat the mushroom caps with olive oil, salt, and black pepper. Lay portobello caps, rounded side up, and burger patties onto the hot grill pan and cook for 5 minutes. Turn the mushroom caps and continue cooking for 1 minute.

Lay a mozzarella slice on top of each patty. Continue cooking until the mushroom caps are softened and the beef patties are no longer pink in the center, 4 to 5 minutes more. Flip the patties and top with cheese. Cook for another 2-3 minutes to be well done while the cheese melts onto the meat. Remove the patties and sandwich them into two mushroom caps each.

Per serving: Cal 505; Fat 39g; Net Carbs 3.2g; Protein 38g

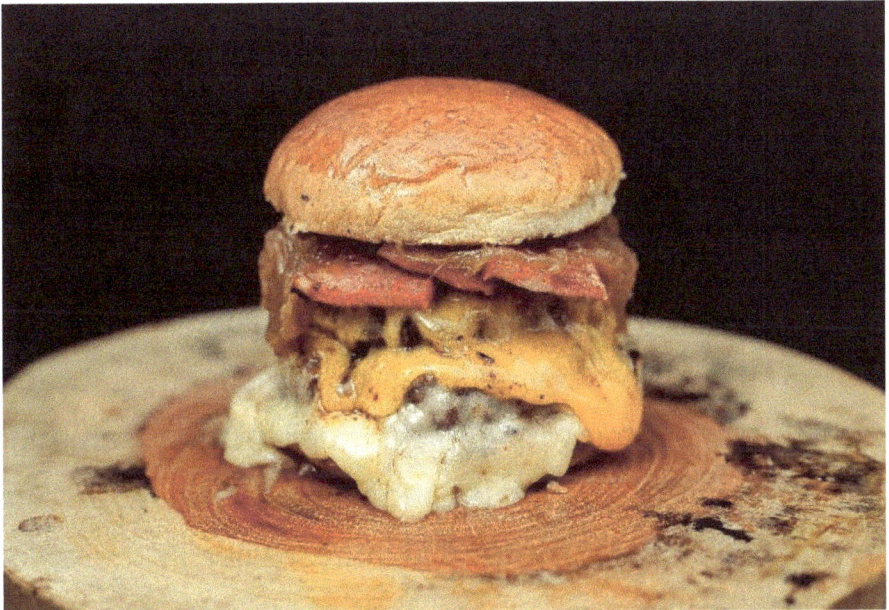

Asian Spiced Beef with Broccoli
Ingredients for 2 servings

½ cup coconut milk

2 tbsp coconut oil

¼ tsp garlic powder

¼ tsp onion powder

½ tbsp coconut aminos

1 lb beef steak, cut into strips

Salt and black pepper to taste

1 head broccoli, cut into florets

½ tbsp Thai green curry paste

1 tsp ginger paste

1 tbsp cilantro, chopped

½ tbsp sesame seeds

Directions and Total Time: approx. 30 minutes

Warm coconut oil in a pan over medium heat, add in the beef, season with garlic powder, pepper, salt, ginger paste, and onion powder and cook for 4 minutes. Mix in broccoli and stir-fry for 5 minutes. Pour in the coconut milk, coconut aminos, and Thai curry paste and cook for 15 minutes. Serve sprinkled with cilantro and sesame seeds.

Per serving: Cal 623; Fat 43g; Net Carbs 2.3g; Protein 53g

Cilantro Beef Balls with Mascarpone

Ingredients for 4 servings

1 garlic clove, minced

1 lb ground beef

1 small onion, chopped

1 jalapeño pepper, chopped

2 tsp cilantro

½ tsp allspice

1 tsp cumin

Salt and black pepper to taste

1 tbsp butter + 1 ½ tbsp melted

½ cup mascarpone cheese

¼ tsp turmeric

¼ tsp baking powder

1 cup flax meal

¼ cup coconut flour

Directions and Total Time: approx. 45 minutes

Puree onion with garlic, jalapeño, and ¼ cup of water in a blender. Melt 1 tbsp butter in a pan over medium heat. Cook the beef for 3 minutes. Stir in the onion mixture, and cook for 2 minutes. Stir in cilantro, salt, cumin, turmeric, allspice, and pepper and cook for 3 minutes.

In a bowl, combine coconut flour, flax meal, and baking powder. In a separate bowl, combine the melted butter with the mascarpone cheese. Combine the 2 mixtures to obtain a dough. Form balls from this mixture, set them on parchment paper, and roll each into a circle.

Split the beef mix on one-half of the dough circles, cover with the other half, seal edges, and lay on a lined sheet. Bake for 25 minutes in the oven at 350 F.

Per serving: Cal 434; Fat 26g; Net Carbs 8.6g; Protein 33g

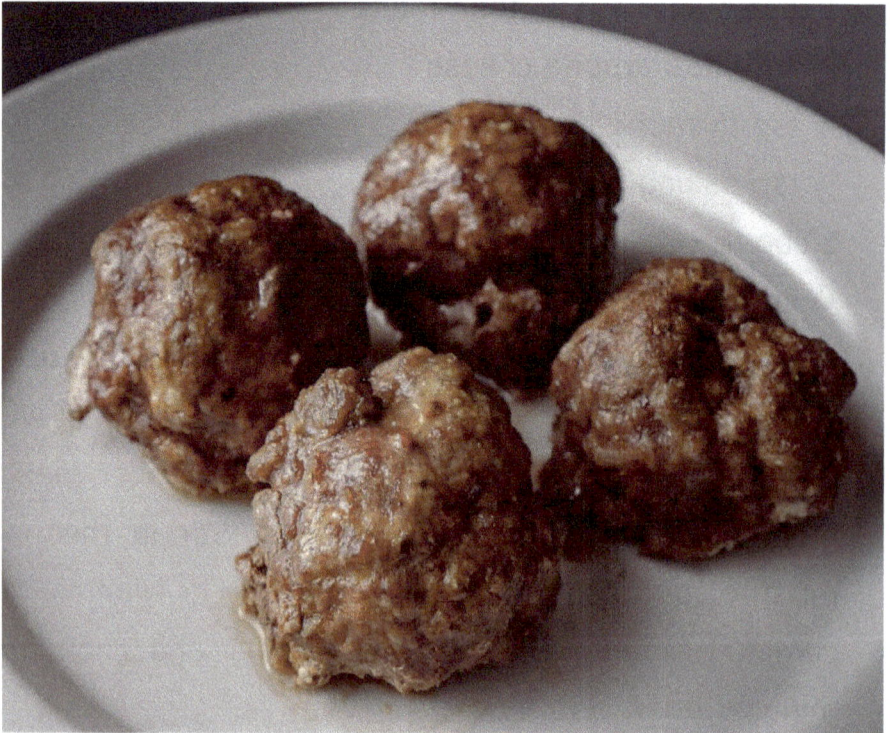

Beef Ragout with Pepper & Green Beans

Ingredients for 4 servings

1 lb chuck steak, trimmed and cubed

2 tbsp olive oil

Salt and black pepper to taste

2 tbsp almond flour

4 green onions, diced

½ cup dry white wine

1 yellow bell pepper, diced

1 cup green beans, chopped

2 tsp Worcestershire sauce

4 oz tomato puree

3 tsp smoked paprika

1 cup beef broth

Parsley leaves to garnish

Directions and Total Time: approx. 2 hours

Dredge the meat in the almond flour and set aside. Place a large skillet over medium heat, add 1 tablespoon of oil to heat and then sauté the green onion, green beans, and bell pepper for 3 minutes. Stir in the paprika and the remaining olive oil. Add the beef and cook for 10 minutes while turning them halfway. Stir in white wine, let it reduce by half, about 3 minutes, and add Worcestershire sauce, tomato puree, and beef broth. Let the mixture boil for 2 minutes, then reduce the heat to lowest and let simmer for 1 ½ hours; stirring now and then. Adjust the taste and dish the ragout. Serve garnished with parsley.

Per serving: Cal 334; Fat 22g; Net Carbs 3.9g; Protein 33g

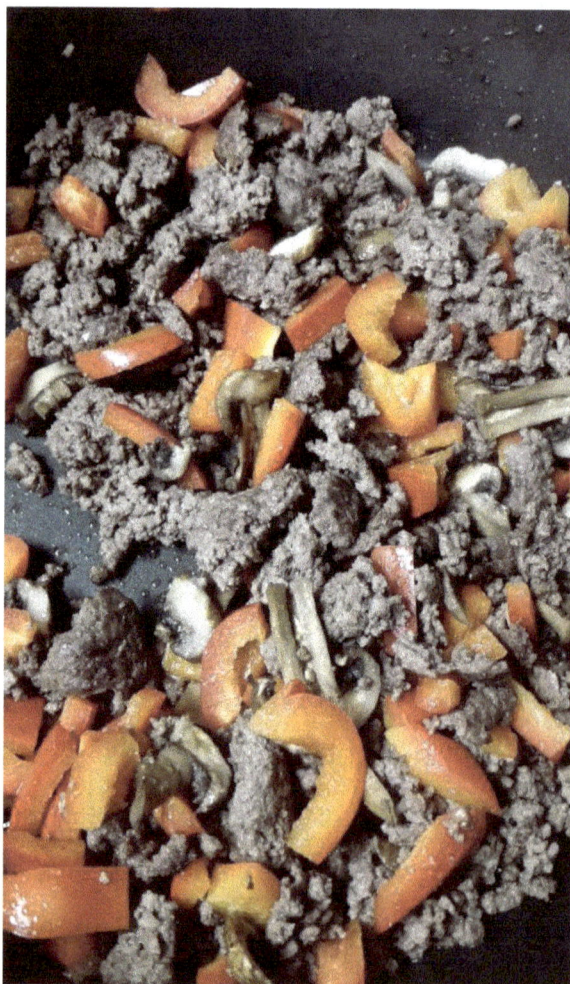

Grilled Beef on Skewers with Fresh Salad

Ingredients for 2 servings

1 lb sirloin steak, boneless, cubed

¼ cup ranch dressing

1 red onion, sliced

½ tbsp white wine vinegar

1 tbsp extra virgin olive oil

2 ripe tomatoes, sliced

2 tbsp fresh parsley, chopped

1 cucumber, sliced

Salt to taste

Directions and Total Time: approx. 20 minutes

Thread the beef cubes on the skewers, about 4 to 5 cubes per skewer. Brush half of the ranch dressing on the skewers (all around).

Preheat grill to high. Place the skewers on the grill and cook for 6 minutes. Turn the skewers and cook further for 6 minutes. Brush the remaining ranch dressing on the meat and cook them for 1 more minute on each side.

In a salad bowl, mix together red onion, tomatoes, and cucumber, sprinkle with salt, vinegar, and extra virgin olive oil; toss to combine. Top the salad with skewers and scatter the parsley all over.

Per serving: Cal 423; Fat 24g; Net Carbs 2.4g; Protein 45g

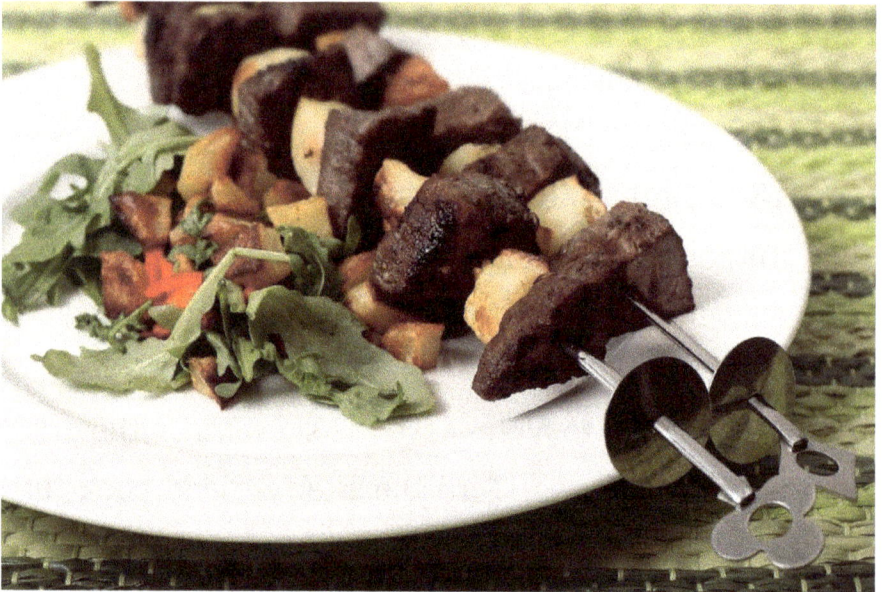

Beef Sausage & Okra Casserole

Ingredients for 4 servings

½ cup marinara sauce, sugar-free

1 cup okra, trimmed

1 tbsp olive oil

1 celery stalk, chopped

¼ cup almond flour

1 egg

1 lb beef sausage, chopped

Salt and black pepper to taste

½ tbsp dried parsley

¼ tsp red pepper flakes

¼ cup Parmesan cheese, grated

2 green onions, chopped

½ tsp garlic powder

¼ tsp dried oregano

½ cup ricotta cheese

1 cup cheddar cheese, grated

Directions and Total Time: approx. 35 minutes

In a bowl, combine the sausage, pepper, pepper flakes, oregano, egg, Parmesan cheese, green onions, almond flour, salt, parsley, celery, and garlic powder. Form balls, lay them on a lined baking sheet, place in the oven at 390 F, and bake for 15 minutes. Remove the balls from the oven and cover with half of the marinara sauce and okra. Pour ricotta cheese all over, followed by the rest of the marinara sauce. Scatter the cheddar cheese and bake in the oven for 10 minutes. Allow to cool before serving.

Per serving: Cal 479; Fat 31g; Net Carbs 4.3g; Protein 39g

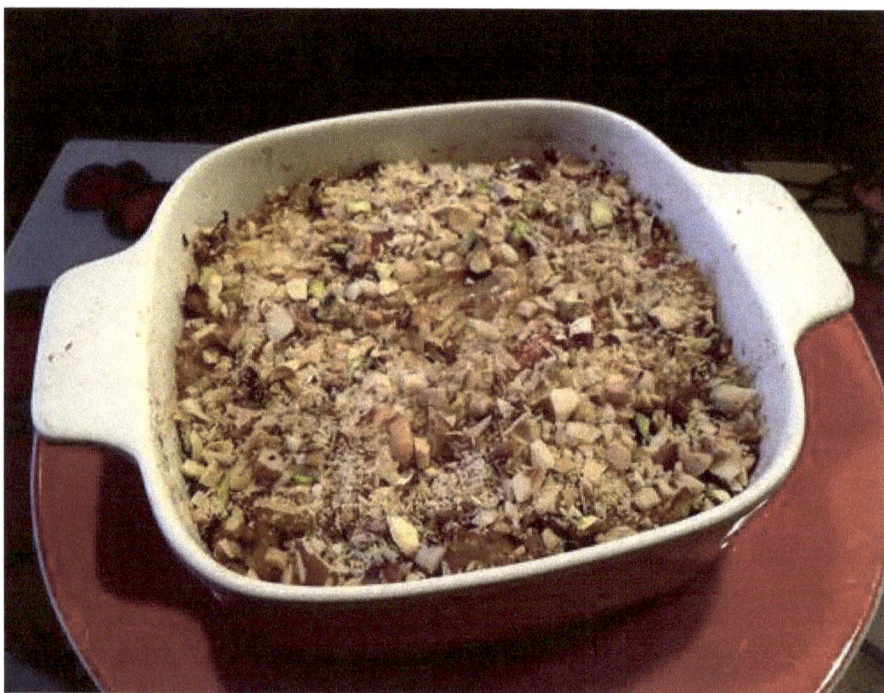

Grilled Beef Steaks & Vegetable Medley
Ingredients for 2 servings

1 red bell pepper, seeded, cut into strips

2 sirloin beef steaks

Salt and black pepper to taste

2 tbsp olive oil

1 ½ tbsp balsamic vinegar

¼ lb asparagus, trimmed

½ cup mushrooms, sliced

½ cup snow peas

1 small onion, quartered

1 garlic clove, sliced

Directions and Total Time: approx. 30 minutes

In a bowl, put asparagus, mushrooms, snow peas, bell pepper, onion, and garlic. Mix salt, pepper, olive oil, and balsamic vinegar in a small bowl, and pour half of the mixture over the vegetables; stir to combine. To the remaining oil mixture, add the beef and toss to coat well.

Preheat a grill pan over high heat. Place the steaks in the grill pan and sear for 6-8 minutes on each side. Remove the beef and set aside. Pour the vegetables and marinade in the pan and cook for 5 minutes, turning once. Share the vegetables into plates. Top with beef and drizzle the sauce from the pan all and serve.

Per serving: Cal 488; Fat 31g; Net Carbs 4.1g; Protein 57g

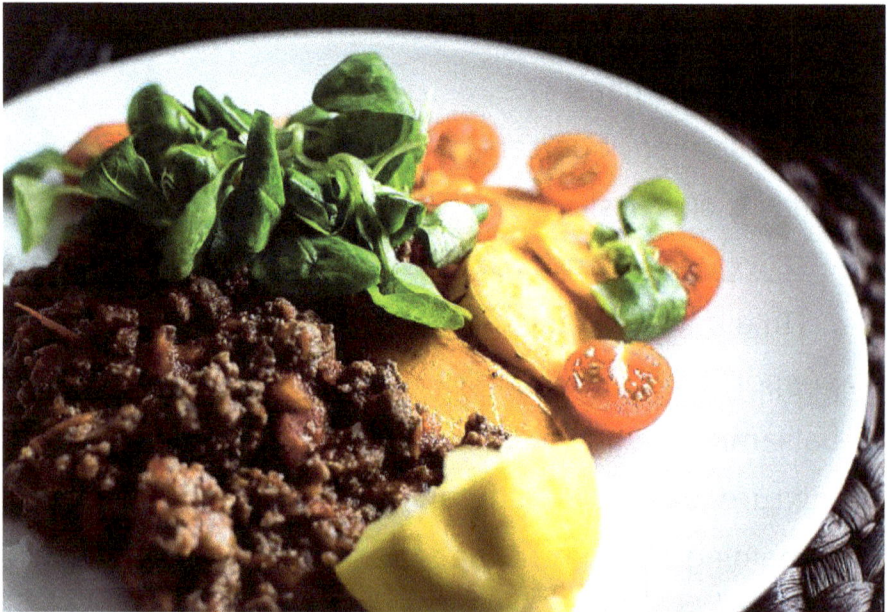

Beef & Mushroom Meatloaf

Ingredients for 4 servings

Meatloaf

1 lb ground beef

½ onion, chopped

1 tbsp almond milk

1 tbsp almond flour

1 garlic clove, minced

1 cup sliced mushrooms

1 small egg

Salt and black pepper to taste

1 tbsp parsley, chopped

⅓ cup Parmesan cheese, grated

Glaze

1/3 cup balsamic vinegar

¼ tbsp xylitol

¼ tsp tomato paste

¼ tsp garlic powder

¼ tsp onion powder

1 tbsp ketchup, sugar-free

Directions and Total Time: approx. 1 hour 10 minutes

Grease a loaf pan with cooking spray and set aside. Preheat oven to 390 F. Combine all meatloaf ingredients in a large bowl. Press this mixture into the prepared loaf pan. Bake in the oven for about 30 minutes. To make the glaze, whisk all ingredients in a bowl. Pour the glaze over the meatloaf. Put the meatloaf back in the oven and cook for 20 more minutes. Let meatloaf sit for 10 minutes before slicing. Serve and enjoy!

Per serving: Cal 311; Fat 21g; Net Carbs 5.5g; Protein 24g

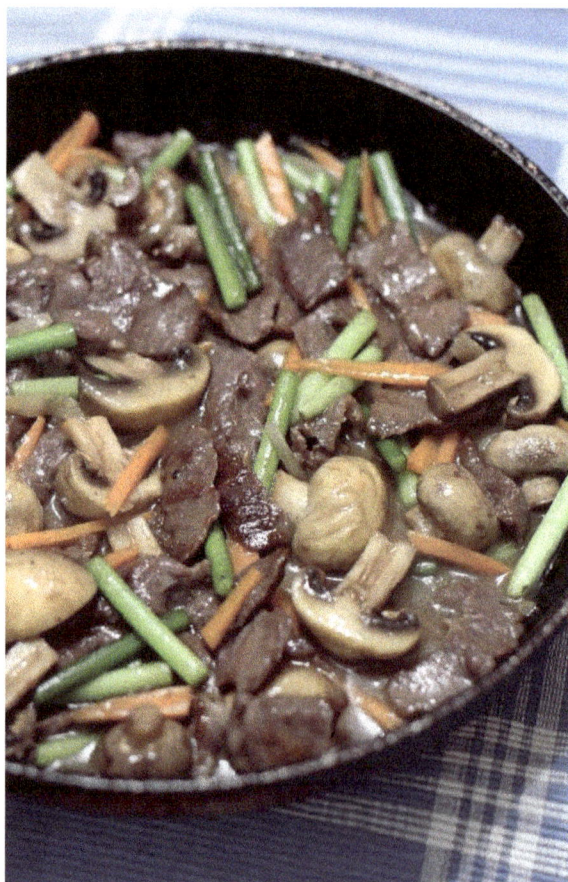

Skirt Steak with Cauli Rice & Green Beans

Ingredients for 4 servings

Hot sauce (sugar-free) for topping

3 cups green beans, chopped

2 cups cauli rice

2 tbsp ghee

1 tbsp olive oil

1 lb skirt steak

Salt and black pepper to taste

4 fresh eggs

Directions and Total Time: approx. 20 minutes

Put the cauli rice and green beans in a bowl. Sprinkle with a little water, and steam in the microwave for 90 seconds to be tender. Share into bowls.

Warm the ghee and olive oil in a skillet, season the beef with salt and black pepper, and brown for 5 minutes on each side. Use a perforated spoon to scoop the meat onto the vegetables. Wipe out the skillet and return to medium heat. Crack in an egg, season with salt and pepper, and cook until the egg white has set, but the yolk is still runny 3 minutes. Remove egg onto the vegetable bowl and fry the remaining 3 eggs. Add to the other bowls. Drizzle with hot sauce and serve.

Per serving: Cal 334; Fat 25g; Net Carbs 6.3g; Protein 14g

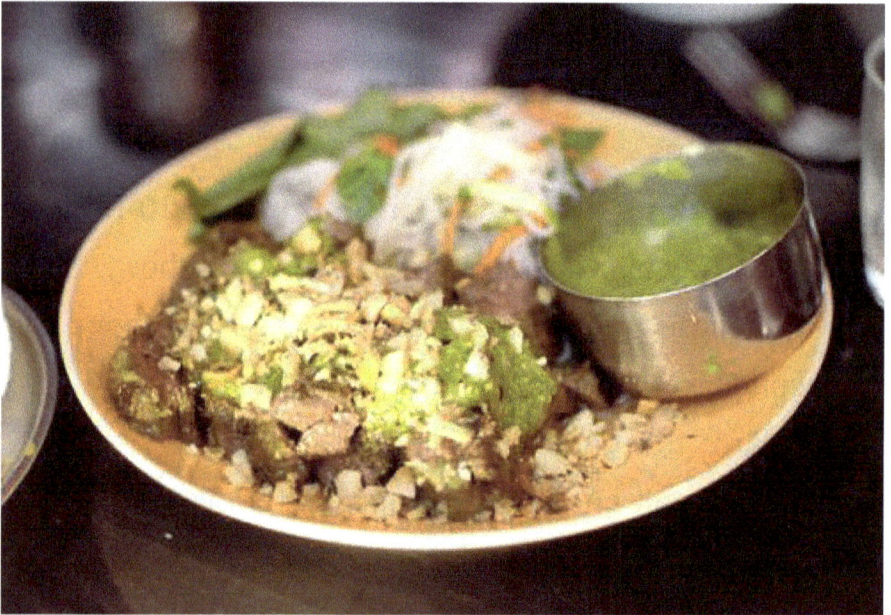

Traditional Scottish Beef with Parsnips
Ingredients for 4 servings

2 tbsp olive oil

12 oz canned corn beef, cubed

1 onion, chopped

4 parsnips, chopped

1 carrot, chopped

1 garlic clove, minced

Salt and black pepper to taste

1 cup vegetable broth

2 tsp rosemary leaves

1 tbsp Worcestershire sauce

½ small cabbage, shredded

Directions and Total Time: approx. 45 minutes

Add the onion, garlic, carrots, rosemary, and parsnips to a warm olive oil over medium heat. Stir and cook for a minute. Pour in the vegetable broth and Worcestershire sauce. Stir the mixture and cook the ingredients on low heat for 25 minutes. Stir in the cabbage and corn beef, season with salt and pepper, and cook for 10 minutes.

Per serving: Cal 321; Fat 16g; Net Carbs 2.3g; Protein 13g

Sunday Beef Gratin
Ingredients for 4 servings

2 tbsp olive oil

1 onion, chopped

1 lb ground beef

2 garlic cloves, minced

Salt and black pepper to taste

1 cup mozzarella, shredded

1 cup fontina cheese, shredded

14 oz canned tomatoes, diced

2 tbsp sesame seeds, toasted

20 dill pickle slices

Directions and Total Time: approx. 35 minutes

Preheat the oven to 390 F. Heat olive oil in a pan over medium heat, place in the beef, garlic, salt, onion, and black pepper, and cook for 5 minutes. Remove and set to a baking dish, stir in half of the tomatoes and mozzarella cheese. Lay the pickle slices on top, spread over the fontina cheese and sesame seeds, and place in the oven to bake for 20 minutes.

Per serving: Cal 523; Fat 43g; Net Carbs 6.5g; Protein 36g

Beef Burgers with Lettuce & Avocado

Ingredients for 2 servings

½ lb ground beef

1 green onion, chopped

½ tsp garlic powder

1 tbsp butter

Salt and black pepper to taste

1 tbsp olive oil

½ tsp Dijon mustard

2 low carb buns, halved

2 tbsp mayonnaise

½ tsp balsamic vinegar

2 tbsp iceberg lettuce, torn

1 avocado, sliced

Directions and Total Time: approx. 15 minutes

In a bowl, mix ground beef, green onion, garlic powder, mustard, salt, and pepper; create 2 burgers. Heat the butter and olive oil in a skillet and cook the burgers for 3 minutes per side. Fill the buns with lettuce, mayonnaise, balsamic vinegar, burgers, and avocado slices to serve.

Per serving: Cal 778; Fat 62g; Net Carbs 5.6g; Protein 34g

Cabbage & Beef Stacks

Ingredients for 4 servings

1 lb chuck steak

1 headcanon cabbage, grated

¼ cup olive oil

3 tbsp coconut flour

1 tsp Italian mixed herb blend

½ cup bone broth

Directions and Total Time: approx. 55 minutes

Preheat the oven to 380 F. Slice the steak thinly across the grain with a sharp knife. In a zipper bag, add coconut flour and beef slices. Seal the bag and shake to coat. Make little mounds of cabbage in a greased baking dish. Drizzle with some olive oil. Remove the beef strips from the coconut flour mixture, shake off the excess flour, and place 2-3 beef strips on each cabbage mound. Sprinkle the Italian herb blend and drizzle again with the remaining olive oil. Roast for 30 minutes. Remove the pan and carefully pour in the broth. Return to the oven and roast further for 10 minutes, until beef cooks through. Serve and enjoy!

Per serving: Cal 231; Net Carbs 1.5g; Fat 14g; Protein 18g

Cauliflower & Beef Casserole

Ingredients for 4 servings

2 tbsp olive oil

1 lb ground beef

Salt and black pepper to taste

½ cup cauli rice

1 tbsp parsley, chopped

1 cup kohlrabi, chopped

5 oz can diced tomatoes

½ cup mozzarella cheese, grated

Directions and Total Time: approx. 40 minutes

Warm the olive oil in a pot over medium heat. Cook the beef for 5-6 minutes until no longer pink, breaking apart with a wooden spatula. Add cauli rice, kohlrabi, tomatoes, and ¼ cup water. Stir and bring to boil covered for 5 minutes to thicken the sauce. Adjust the taste with salt and black pepper. Spoon the beef mixture into the baking dish and spread evenly. Sprinkle with mozzarella cheese. Bake in the oven for 15 minutes at 380 F until the cheese has melted and it's golden brown. Remove and cool for 4 minutes. Serve sprinkled with parsley.

Per serving: Cal 391; Fat 233g; Net Carbs 7.3g; Protein 20g

Spiralized Zucchini in Bolognese Sauce
Ingredients for 4 servings

4 zucchinis, spiralized

1 lb ground beef

2 bacon slices, chopped

2 garlic cloves

1 onion, chopped

1 tsp dried oregano

1 tsp sage

1 tsp rosemary

7 oz canned diced tomatoes

2 tbsp olive oil

Directions and Total Time: approx. 35 minutes

Cook the zoodles in warm olive oil over medium heat for 3-4 minutes and remove to a serving plate. To the same pan, add bacon, onion, and garlic and cook for 3 minutes. Add beef and cook until browned, about 4-5 minutes. Stir in the herbs and tomatoes. Cook for 15 minutes and serve over the zoodles.

Per serving: Cal 378; Fat 19g; Net Carbs 5.9g; Protein 41g

Juicy Beef with Rosemary & Thyme

Ingredients for 4 servings

2 garlic cloves, minced

2 tbsp butter

2 tbsp olive oil

1 tbsp rosemary, chopped

1 lb beef rump steak, sliced

Salt and black pepper to taste

1 shallot, chopped

½ cup heavy cream

½ cup beef stock

1 tbsp mustard

2 tsp soy sauce, sugar-free

2 tsp lemon juice

1 tsp xylitol

A sprig of rosemary

A sprig of thyme

Directions and Total Time: approx. 30 minutes

Set a pan to medium heat, warm in a tbsp of olive oil and stir in the shallot; cook for 3 minutes. Stir in the stock, soy sauce, xylitol, thyme sprig, cream, mustard and rosemary sprig, and cook for 8 minutes. Stir in butter, lemon juice, pepper and salt. Get rid of the rosemary and thyme. Set aside. In a bowl, combine the remaining oil with black pepper, garlic, rosemary, and salt. Toss in the beef to coat, and set aside for some minutes.

Heat a pan over medium-high heat, place in the beef steak, cook for 6 minutes, flipping halfway through; set aside and keep warm. Plate the beef slices, sprinkle over the sauce, and enjoy.

Per serving: Cal 411; Fat 31g; Net Carbs 4.6g; Protein 28g

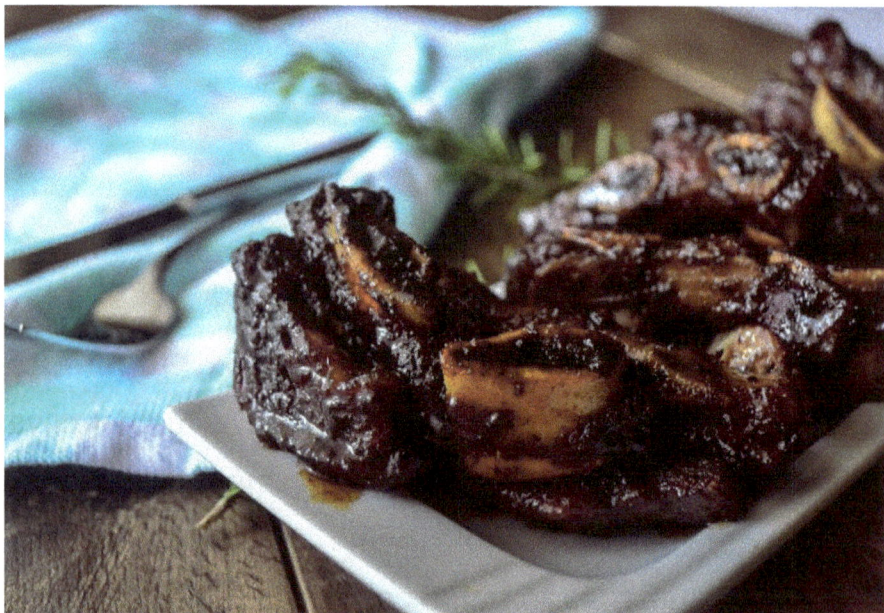

Red Wine Beef Roast with Vegetables

Ingredients for 2 servings

1 tbsp olive oil

1 lb brisket

½ cup carrots, peeled

1 red onion, quartered

2 stalks celery, cut into chunks

1 garlic clove, minced

Salt and black pepper to taste

1 bay leaf

1 tbsp fresh thyme, chopped

1 cup red wine

Directions and Total Time: approx. 2 hours 20 minutes

Season the brisket with salt and pepper. Brown the meat on both sides in warm olive oil over medium heat for 6-8 minutes. Transfer to a deep casserole dish. Arrange the carrots, onion, garlic, thyme, celery, and bay leaf around the brisket and pour in the red wine and ½ cup of water. Cover the pot and place in the preheated to 370 F oven.

Cook for 2 hours. When ready, remove the casserole. Transfer the beef to a chopping board and cut it into thick slices. Top the beef with vegetables to serve.

Per serving: Cal 446; Fat 22g; Net Carbs 5.6g; Protein 52g

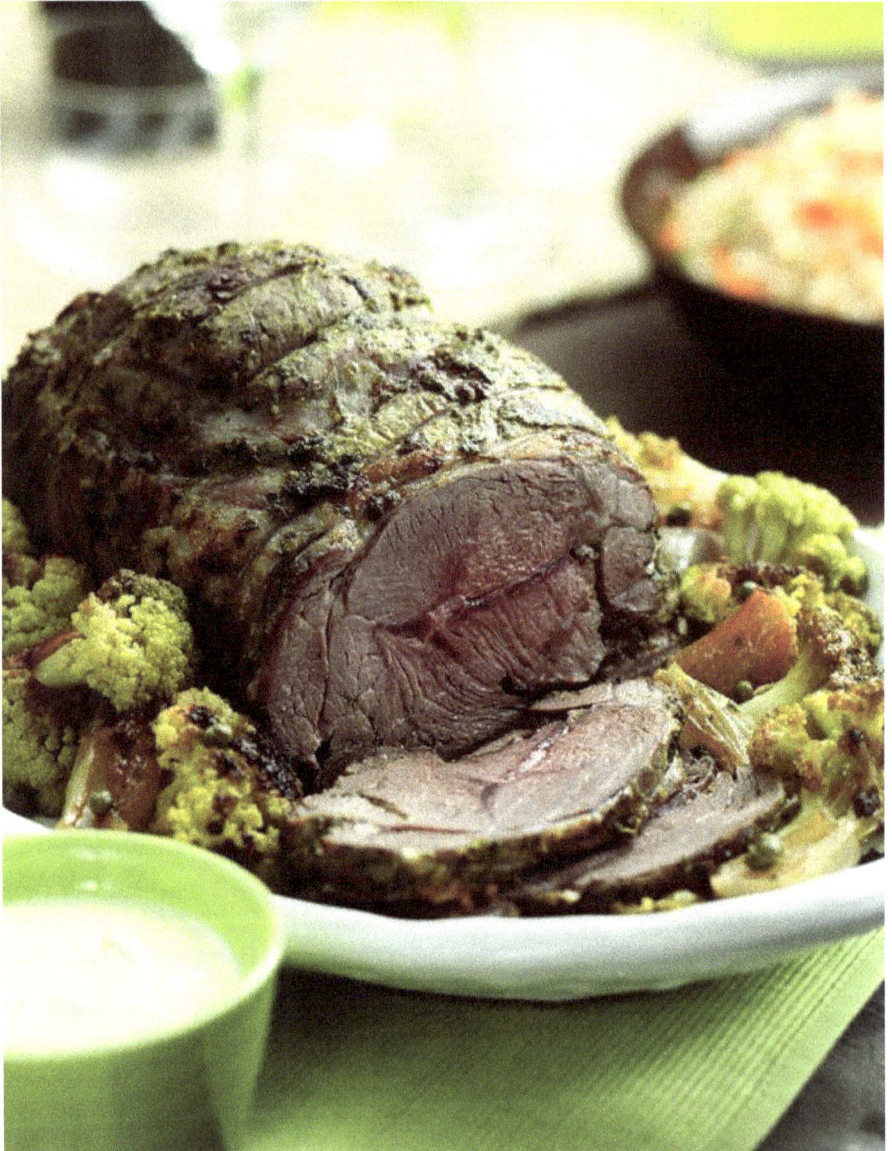

Grilled Steak with Green Beans
Ingredients for 2 servings

2 rib-eye steaks

2 tbsp unsalted butter

1 tsp olive oil

½ cup green beans, sliced

Salt and black pepper to taste

1 tbsp fresh thyme, chopped

1 tbsp rosemary, chopped

1 tbsp fresh parsley, chopped

Directions and Total Time: approx. 20 minutes

Preheat a grill pan over high heat. Brush the steaks with olive oil and season with salt and black pepper. Cook the steaks for about 4 minutes per side; reserve. Steam the green beans for 3-4 minutes until tender.

Season with salt. Melt the butter in the pan and stir-fry the herbs for 1 minute; then mix in the green beans. Place over the steaks and serve. Enjoy!

Per serving: Cal 576; Fat 39g; Net Carbs 4.3g; Protein 51g

Eggplant Beef Lasagna
Ingredients for 4 servings

2 large eggplants, sliced lengthwise

2 tbsp olive oil

½ red chili, chopped

1 lb ground beef

2 garlic cloves, minced

1 shallot, chopped

1 cup tomato sauce

Salt and black pepper to taste

2 tsp sweet paprika

1 tsp dried thyme

1 tsp dried basil

1 cup mozzarella cheese, grated

1 cup chicken broth

Directions and Total Time: approx. 65 minutes

Heat the oil in a skillet and cook the beef for 4 minutes while breaking any lumps as you stir. Top with shallot, garlic, chili, tomato sauce, salt, paprika and black pepper. Stir and cook for 5 more minutes.

Lay 1/3 of the eggplant slices in a greased baking dish. Top with 1/3 of the beef mixture and repeat the layering process two more times with the same quantities. Season with basil and thyme. Pour in the chicken broth. Sprinkle the mozzarella cheese on top and tuck the baking dish in the oven. Bake for 35 minutes at 380 F. Remove the lasagna and let it rest for 10 minutes before serving.

Per serving: Cal 388; Fat 16g; Net Carbs 9.8g; Protein 41g

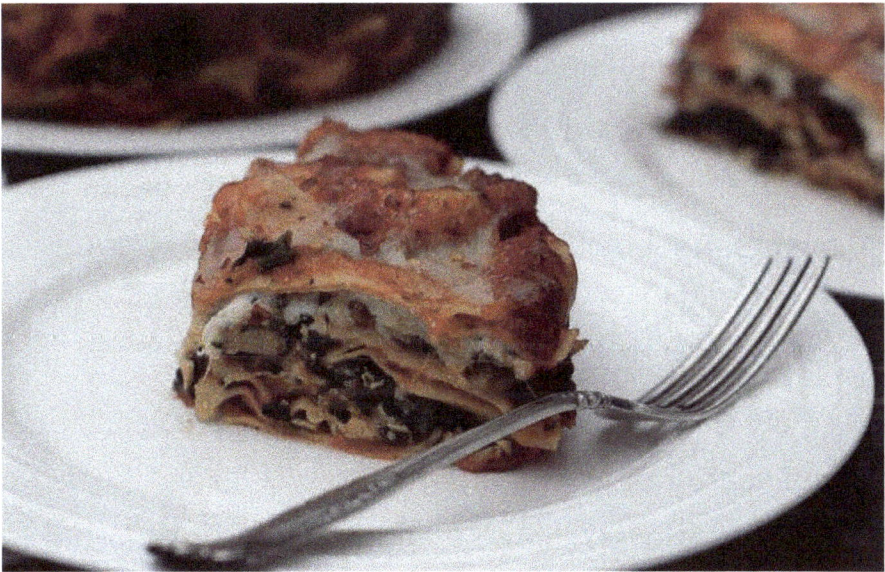

Beef Steaks with Bacon & Mushrooms

Ingredients for 2 servings

2 oz bacon, chopped

1 cup mushrooms, sliced

1 garlic clove, chopped

1 shallot, chopped

1 cup heavy cream

½ lb beef steaks

1 tsp ground nutmeg

¼ cup coconut oil

Salt and black pepper to taste

1 tbsp parsley, chopped

Directions and Total Time: approx. 50 minutes

In a pan over medium heat, cook the bacon for 2-3 minutes; set aside. In the same pan, warm the oil, add in the shallot, garlic and mushrooms. Cook for 4 minutes .

Stir in the beef, season with salt, pepper, and nutmeg, and sear until browned, 2 minutes per side.

Preheat oven to 360 F and insert the pan in the oven to bake for 25 minutes. Remove the beef steaks to a bowl and cover with foil. Place the pan over medium heat, pour in the heavy cream over the mushroom mixture, add in the reserved bacon and cook for 5 minutes; remove from heat. Spread the bacon/mushroom sauce over beef steaks, sprinkle with parsley and serve.

Per serving: Cal 765; Fat 71g; Net Carbs 3.8g; Protein 32g

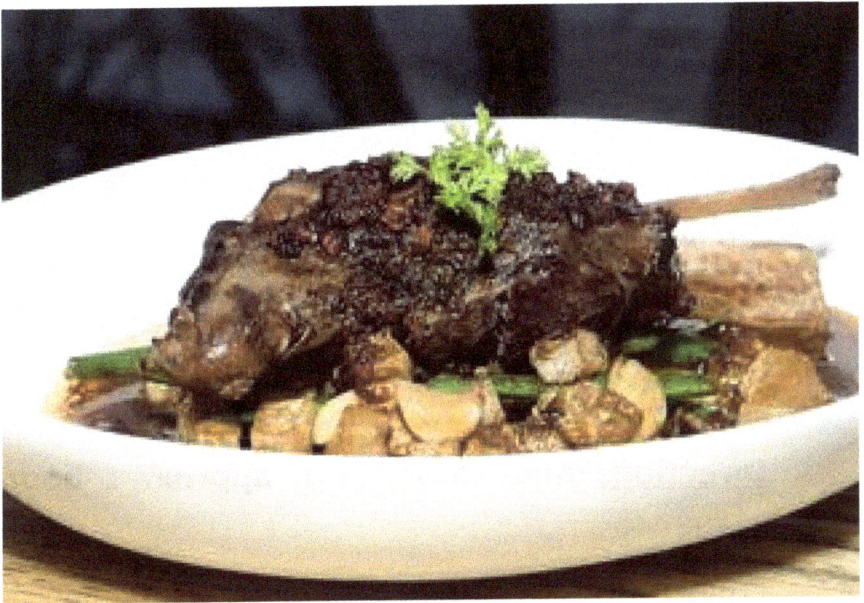

Veggie Chuck Roast Beef in Oven
Ingredients for 4 servings

2 tbsp olive oil

1 lb beef chuck roast, cubed

1 cup canned diced tomatoes

1 carrot, chopped

Salt and black pepper to taste

½ lb mushrooms, sliced

1 celery stalk, chopped

1 bell pepper, sliced

1 onion, chopped

1 bay leaf

½ cup beef stock

1 tbsp rosemary, chopped

½ tsp dry mustard

1 tbsp almond flour

Directions and Total Time: approx. 1 hour 45 minutes

Preheat oven to 350 F. Set a pot over medium heat, warm olive oil and brown the beef on each side for 4-5 minutes. Stir in tomatoes, onion, mustard, carrot, mushrooms, bell pepper, celery, bay leaf, and stock. Season with salt and pepper. In a bowl, combine ½ cup of water with flour and stir in the pot. Transfer to a baking dish and bake for 90 minutes, stirring at intervals of 30 minutes. Scatter the rosemary over and serve warm.

Per serving: Cal 325; Fat 18g; Net Carbs 5.6g; Protein 31g

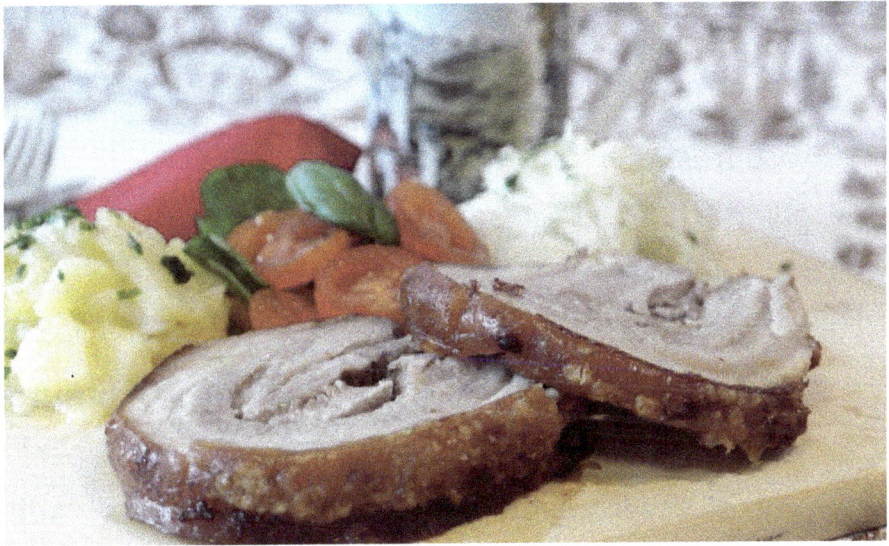

Winter Beef Stew

Ingredients for 4 servings

14 oz canned tomatoes with juice

3 tsp olive oil

1 lb ground beef

1 cup beef stock

1 carrot, chopped

1 celery stick, chopped

1 lb butternut squash, diced

1 tbsp Worcestershire sauce

2 bay leaves

Salt and black pepper to taste

3 tbsp fresh parsley, chopped

1 onion, chopped

1 tsp dried sage

1 garlic clove, minced

Directions and Total Time: approx. 40 minutes

Cook the onion, garlic, celery, carrot, and beef, in warm oil over medium heat for 10 minutes. Add in butternut squash, Worcestershire sauce, bay leaves, stock, canned tomatoes, and sage, and bring to a boil. Reduce heat and simmer for 20 minutes. Adjust the seasonings. Remove and discard the bay leaves. Serve topped with parsley.

Per serving: Cal 353; Fat 16g; Net Carbs 6.6g; Protein 26g

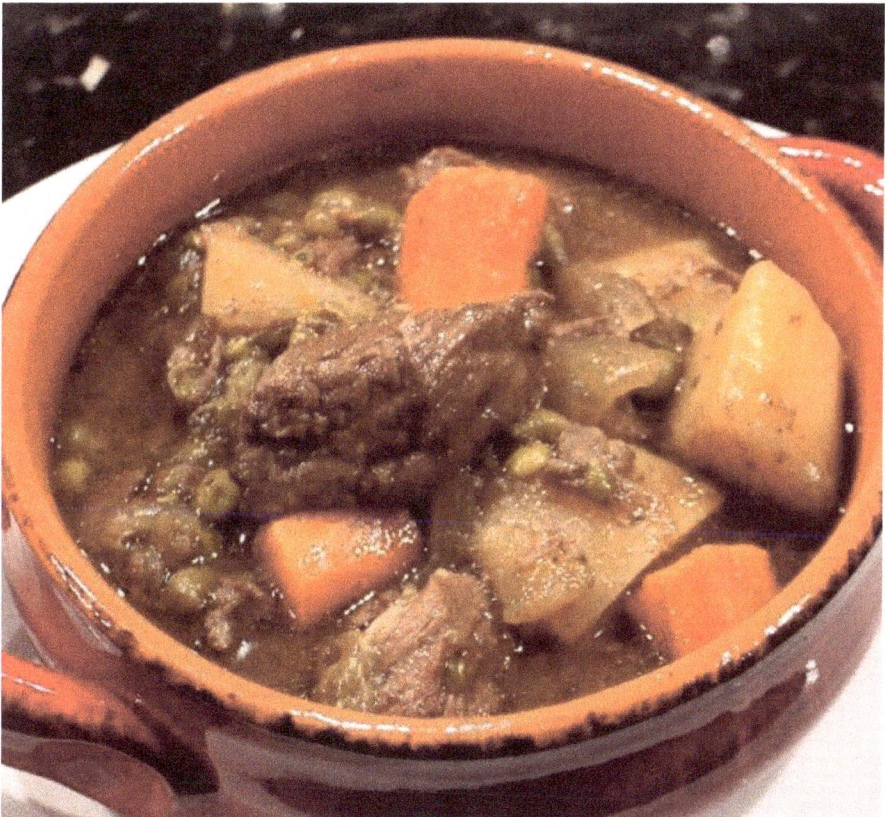

Beef Cheese & Egg Casserole

Ingredients for 4 servings

2 tbsp olive oil

½ tsp nutmeg

1 lb ground beef

5 eggs, beaten

1 cup Gouda cheese, grated

1 yellow onion, chopped

2 cups tomatoes, chopped

¼ cup heavy cream

1 Banana pepper, chopped

2 garlic cloves, chopped

2 zucchinis, sliced

Salt and black pepper to taste

Directions and Total Time: approx. 25 minutes

Preheat oven to 360 F. Warm the olive oil in a skillet over medium heat. Stir-fry the garlic, banana pepper, and onion for 2 minutes until tender. Add the ground beef and sauté for 4-6 minutes, stirring often.

Sprinkle with nutmeg, salt, and pepper. Transfer the mixture to a baking dish. Cover with tomatoes and arrange the zucchini slices on top. Bake for 30 minutes.

In a bowl, mix the eggs, cheese, and heavy cream. Season with salt and pepper. Remove the baking dish from the oven and pour the cheese mixture over. Bake for 10-15 more minutes or until the eggs are set. Enjoy!

Per serving: Cal 608; Net Carbs 8.4g; Fat 36g; Protein 56g

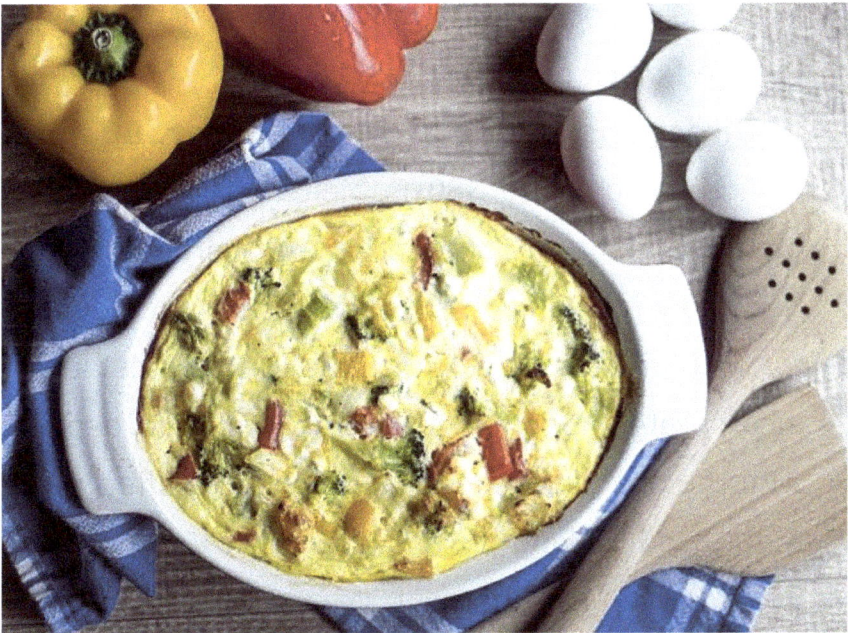

Bell Peppers Stuffed with Enchilada Beef
Ingredients for 6 servings

3 tbsp butter, softened

6 bell peppers, deseeded

½ white onion, chopped

3 cloves garlic, minced

2 ½ lb ground beef

3 tsp enchilada seasoning

1 cup cauliflower rice

¼ cup grated cheddar cheese

Sour cream for serving

Salt and black pepper to taste

Directions and Total Time: approx. 60 minutes

Preheat oven to 380 F. Melt butter in a skillet over medium heat and sauté onion and garlic for 3 minutes. Stir in beef, enchilada seasoning, salt, and pepper. Cook for 10 minutes. Mix in the cauli rice until well incorporated. Spoon the mixture into the peppers, top with the cheddar cheese, and put the stuffed peppers in a greased baking dish. Bake for 40 minutes. Drop generous dollops of sour cream on the peppers and serve.

Per serving: Cal 411; Net Carbs 4g; Fat 19g; Protein 48g

Lettuce Cups with Spicy Beef
Ingredients for 4 servings

3 tbsp ghee, divided

1 lb chuck steak

1 large white onion, chopped

2 garlic cloves, minced

1 jalapeño pepper, chopped

2 tsp red curry powder

1 cup cauliflower rice

8 small lettuce leaves

Salt and black pepper to taste

¼ cup sour cream for topping

Directions and Total Time: approx. 30 minutes

Warm 2 tbsp of the ghee in a large deep skillet. Sliced the beef thinly against the grain and cook until brown and cooked within, 10 minutes; set aside. Sauté the onion in the skillet for 3 minutes. Pour in garlic, salt, pepper, and jalapeño and cook for 1 minute.

Add the remaining ghee, curry powder, and beef. Cook for 5 minutes and stir in the cauliflower rice. Sauté until adequately mixed and the cauliflower is slightly softened, 2 to 3 minutes. Adjust the taste with salt and pepper.

Lay out the lettuce leaves on a lean flat surface and spoon the beef mixture onto the middle part of them, 3 tbsp per leaf. Top with sour cream, wrap the leaves, and serve.

Per serving: Cal 302; Net Carbs 3.3g; Fat 21g; Protein 32g

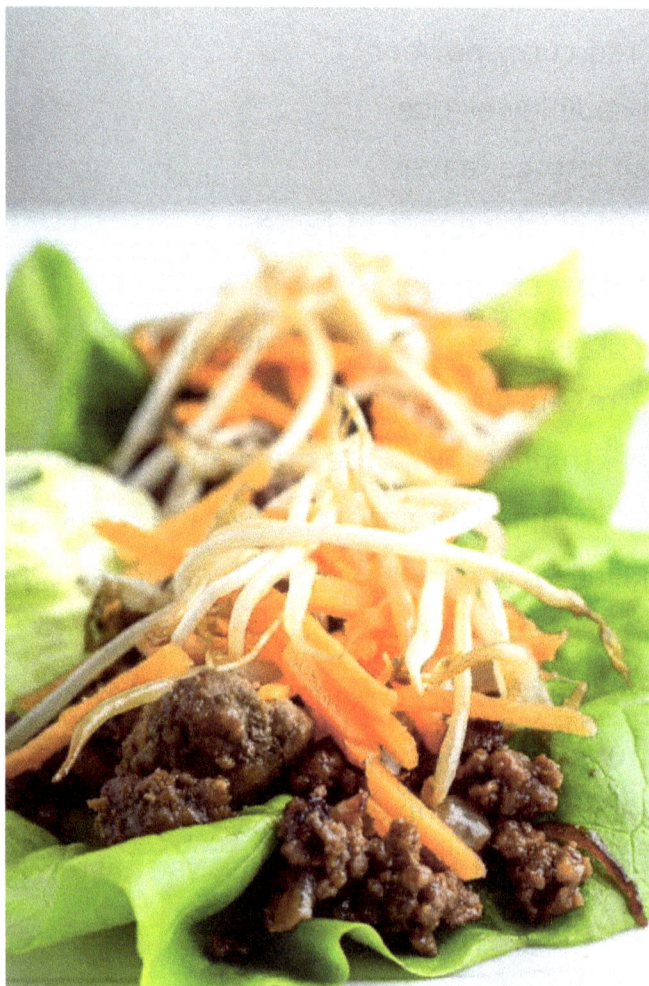

Basil Beef Sausage Pizza

Ingredients for 4 servings

2 tbsp butter

2 tbsp cream cheese, softened

10 oz shredded mozzarella

8 oz ground beef sausage

1 egg

¾ cup almond flour

1 tsp plain vinegar

¼ cup tomato sauce

½ tsp dried basil

Directions and Total Time: approx. 50 minutes

Preheat oven to 390 F. Line a pizza pan with parchment paper. Melt the cream cheese and half of the mozzarella cheese in a skillet over low heat while stirring until evenly combined. Turn the heat off and mix in almond flour, egg, and vinegar. Let cool slightly.

Flatten the mixture onto the pizza pan. Cover with another parchment paper and, using a rolling pin, smoothen the dough into a circle. Take off the parchment paper on top, prick the dough all over with a fork and bake for 10 to 15 minutes until golden brown.

While the crust bakes, melt butter in a skillet over and fry sausage until brown, 8 minutes. Turn the heat off.

Spread the tomato sauce on the crust, top with basil, meat, and remaining mozzarella cheese, and return to the oven. Bake for 12 minutes. Remove the pizza, slice, and serve.

Per serving: Cal 359; Net Carbs 0.8g; Fat 19g; Protein 41g

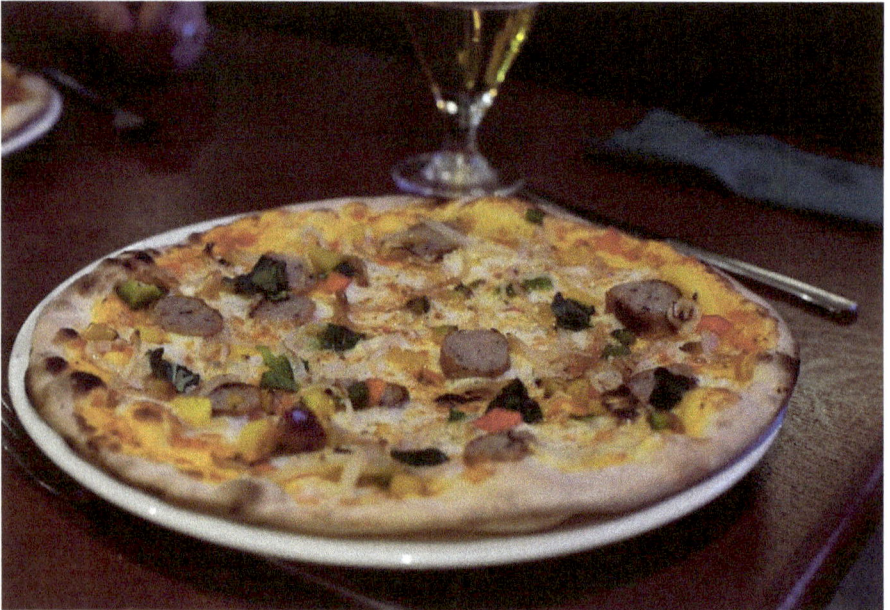

Spinach Cheeseburgers

Ingredients for 4 servings

1 lb ground beef

4 tomato wedges, deseeded

½ cup chopped cilantro

1 lemon, zested and juiced

1 tsp garlic powder

2 tbsp hot chili puree

16 large spinach leaves

4 tbsp mayonnaise

1 medium red onion, sliced

¼ cup grated Parmesan

1 avocado, halved, sliced

Salt and black pepper to taste

Directions and Total Time: approx. 15 minutes

Preheat the grill to high heat. In a bowl, add beef, cilantro, lemon zest, juice, salt, pepper, garlic powder, and chili puree. Mix the ingredients until evenly combined.

Make 4 patties from the mixture. Grill for 3 minutes per side. Transfer to a serving plate. Lay 2 spinach leaves side to side in 4 portions on a clean flat surface. Place a beef patty on each and spread 1 tbsp of mayo on top. Add a slice of tomato and onion, sprinkle with some

Parmesan, and place avocado on top. Cover with 2 pieces of spinach leaves each. Serve the burgers with cream cheese sauce.

Per serving: Cal 308; Net Carbs 6.5g; Fat 16g; Protein 31g

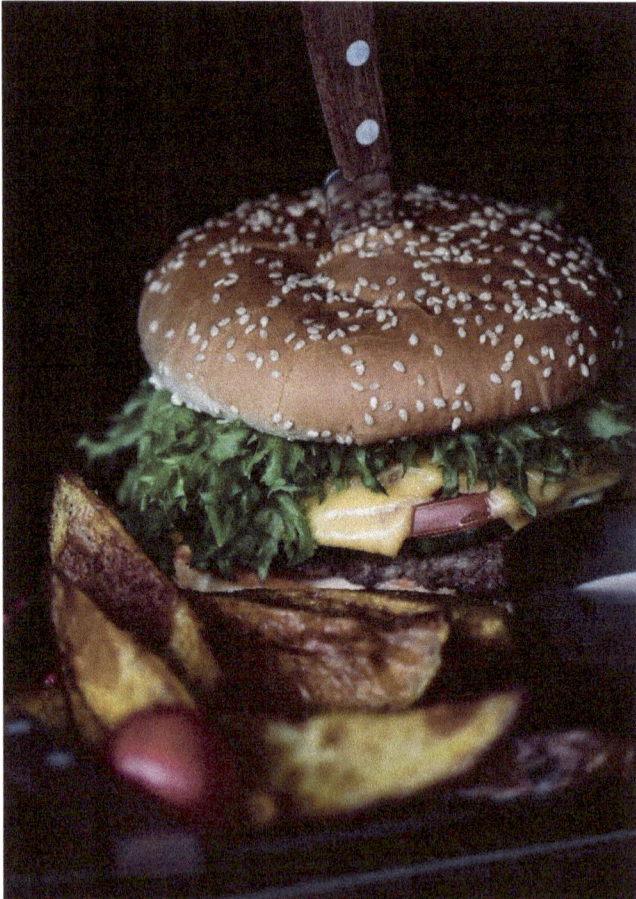

Beef Pad Thai with Peanuts & Zucchini
Ingredients for 4 servings

3 large eggs, lightly beaten

2 ½ lb chuck steak

1 tsp red pepper flakes

1 tsp pureed garlic

¼ tsp freshly ground ginger

2 tbsp peanut oil

3 ¼ tbsp peanut butter

1/3 cup beef broth

2 tbsp tamari sauce

1 tbsp white vinegar

½ cup chopped green onions

2 garlic cloves, minced

4 zucchinis, spiralized

½ cup bean sprouts

½ cup crushed peanuts

Salt and black pepper to taste

Directions and Total Time: approx. 30 minutes

Using a sharp knife, slice the beef thinly against the grain. In a bowl, combine garlic puree, ginger, salt, and pepper. Add in beef and toss to coat.

Heat peanut oil in a deep skillet and cook the beef for 12 minutes; transfer to a plate. Pour the eggs into the skillet and scramble for 1 minute; set aside. Reduce the heat and combine broth, peanut butter, tamari sauce, vinegar, green onions, minced garlic, and red pepper flakes.

Mix until adequately combined and simmer for 3 minutes. Stir in beef, zucchini, bean sprouts, and eggs. Cook for 1 minute. Garnish with peanuts.

Per serving: Cal 433; Net Carbs 3.3g; Fat 38g; Protein 69g

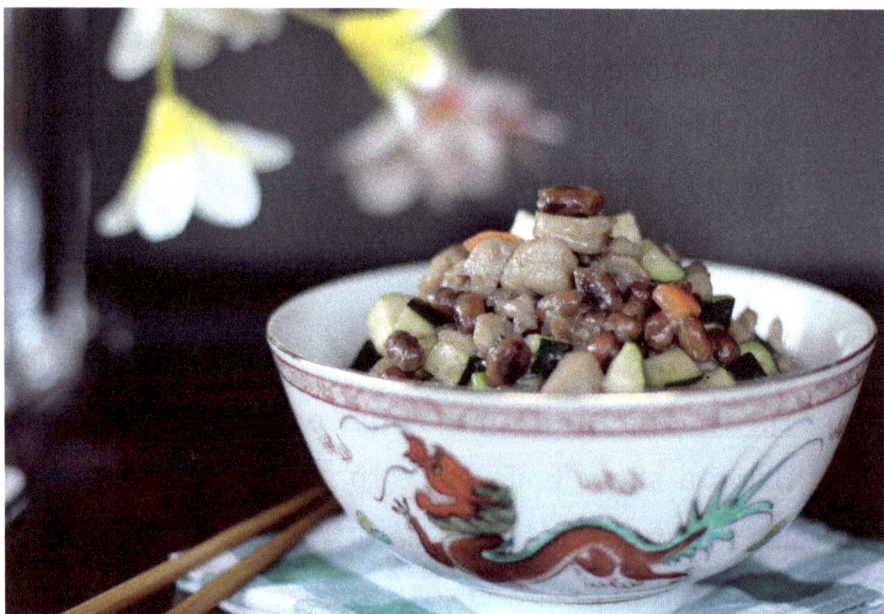

Chicken With Coconut Curry
Macros: Fat 71% | Protein 22% | Carbs 7%

Prep time: 20 minutes | Cook time: 30 minutes | Serves 6

This flavorful chicken with keto coconut curry recipe is EASY, with a secret trick! You are only 9 ingredients away from low-carbon coconut curry, and 30 minutes away. The easy chicken curry will be a family-wide dinner winner. Plus, it is gluten-free and keto-friendly.

2 stalks of lemongrass

1½ pounds (680 g) boneless chicken thighs

2 tablespoons coconut oil

1 tablespoon curry powder

1 thumb-sized piece of fresh ginger

Salt and freshly ground black pepper, to taste

1 leek

2 garlic cloves

1 small red bell pepper, sliced

½ red chili pepper, finely chopped

14 ounces (397 g) coconut cream

1 lemon, zest

1. Crush the rough part of the lemongrass with the broad side of a knife or a pestle.

2. Cut the chicken into coarse pieces.

3. Gently heat the coconut oil in a wok or a large frying pan.

4. Grate the ginger and fry together with the lemongrass and curry.

5. Add half of the chicken and sauté over medium heat until the strips are golden. Salt and pepper to taste.

6. Set aside and fry the rest of the chicken in the same way, perhaps add a little more curry for the second batch. The lemon grass can remain in the pan.

7. Slice the leek into pieces and sauté them in the same pan together with the other vegetables and the finely chopped garlic. The vegetables should turn golden, but retain their crispiness.

8. Add the coconut cream and chicken and let simmer for 5 to 10 minutes until everything is warm.

9. Remove the lemon grass and sprinkle over the lime zest.

STORAGE: Keep your leftovers well sealed and separate. Keeping foods separate and well covered helps to combat potential cross-contamination. store it in a glass or plastic container or to save room for 4 days in the fridge and for 1 month in the freezer, put it into a freezer bag and lay it flat so that it freezes flat.

REHEAT: Microwave, covered, or reheated in a frying pan or instant pot, covered, on medium until the desired temperature is reached. Don't reheat leftovers more than once. This is because the more times you cool and reheat food, the higher the risk of food poisoning.

SERVE IT WITH: Serve with keto eggplant salad with capsicum and a glass of fresh juice.

PER SERVING

calories: 578 | fat: 46.6g | total carbs: 10.8g | fiber: 2.8g | protein: 32.6g

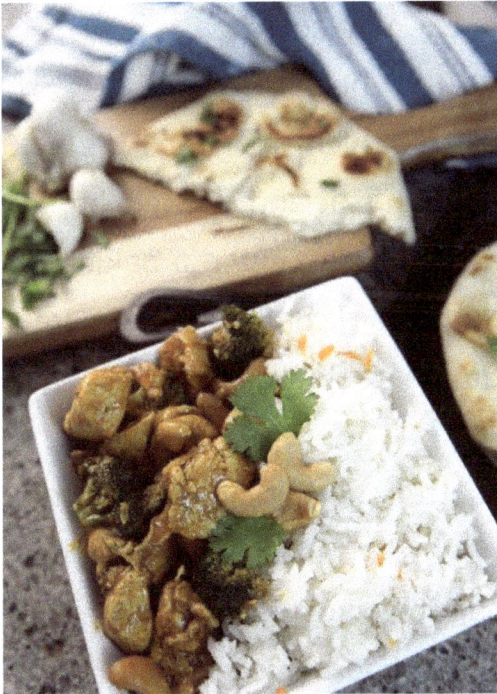

Oven-Baked Chicken in Garlic
Macros: Fat 56% | Protein 43% | Carbs 0%

Prep time: 10 minutes | Cook time: 55 minutes | Serves 4

Looking for a one-pan meal with your family? Or maybe you're just looking for a meal with easy preparation? This oven-baked keto chicken in garlic just needs a big baking dish. It is beautifully flavorful and fragrant. Who knew that a chicken dish would fit into a diet so well?

3 pounds (1.4 kg) chicken

2 teaspoons sea salt

½ teaspoon ground black pepper

2 garlic cloves, minced

6 ounces (170 g) butter

1. Preheat the oven to 400°F (205°C). Season the chicken with salt and pepper, both inside and out.

2. Place chicken breast up in a baking dish.

3. Combine the garlic and butter in a small saucepan over medium heat. The butter should not turn brown, just melt.

4. Let the butter cool for a couple of minutes.

5. Pour the garlic butter over and inside the chicken. Bake on lower oven rack for 1-1 ½ hours, or until internal temperature reaches 180°F (82°C). Baste

with the juices from the bottom of the pan every 20 minutes.

6. Serve with th e juices and a side dish of your choice.

STORAGE: Keeping foods separate and well covered helps to combat potential cross-contamination. store it in a plastic container in the fridge for up to 3 to 4 days or in the freezer for up to 3 weeks

REHEAT: Microwave, covered, or reheated in a frying pan or instant pot, covered, on medium until the desired temperature is reached. Don't reheat leftovers more than once. This is because the more times you cool and reheat food, the higher the risk of food poisoning.

SERVE IT WITH: Serve with salad or steamed low-carb vegetables and a glass of fresh juice.

PER SERVING

calories: 686 | fat: 43.7g | total carbs: 0.8g | fiber: 0.1g | protein: 69.7g

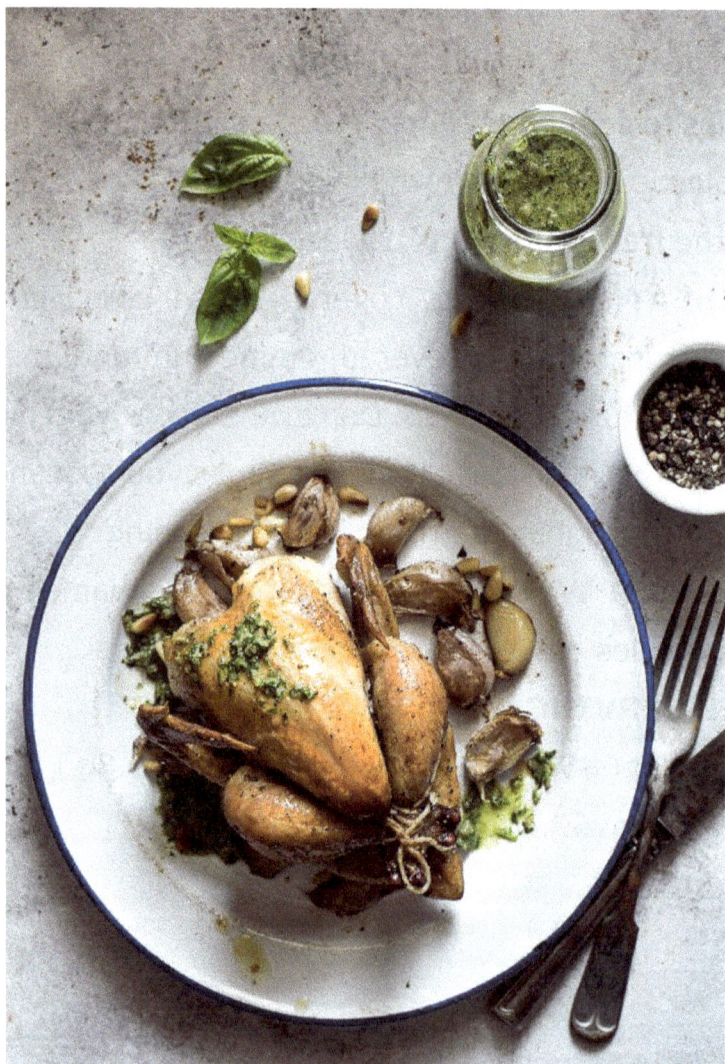

Chubby And Juicy Roasted Chicken
Macros: Fat 64% | Protein 34% | Carbs 2%

Prep time: 15 minutes | Cook time: 45 minutes | Serves 4

Thinking of the perfect dish for your special occasion or a simple dinner with the family, palmy roasted chicken is always a crowd-pleaser. Butter, garlic, and lemon give the chicken a rich flavor, while it's cooked away with healthy, aromatic butter or olive oil. Lemon and garlic are just such a wonderful combination!

1 teaspoon olive oil

1 lemon, zested and cut in half

½ tablespoon ground cinnamon

½ tablespoon ground ginger

3 sprigs fresh thyme, chopped

2 sprigs fresh rosemary, chopped

2 cloves garlic, minced

Sea salt and freshly ground black pepper, to taste

1 (3-pound / 1.4-kg) whole chicken

4 whole garlic cloves

¾ cup water

1. Preheat the oven to 400°F (205°C).

2. In a bowl, mix together the olive oil, lemon zest, cinnamon, ginger, rosemary, thyme, and minced garlic. To taste, add a pinch salt and pepper.

3. Rub ⅔ of the mixture over the meat under the skin of the chicken. Stuff the cavity with half of the lemon along with the 4 garlic cloves. This will render the chicken a delicious flavor.

4. Rub the remaining mixture over the outside of the chicken and season with salt and pepper.

5. Arrange the chicken in a roasting pan and pour ¾ cup of water into the pan, Squeeze the juice from the remaining lemon half and rub evenly over the chicken.

6. Place the chicken in the preheated oven for 45 minutes until completely cooked through and an instant-read thermometer inserted into the thickest part of the thigh, near the bone registers at least 165°F (74°C).

7. Remove from the oven and cover the pan with a doubled sheet of aluminum foil. Let rest for 5 to 10 minutes before serving.

STORAGE: Store in an airtight container in the fridge for up to 4 days or in the freezer for up to 1 month.

REHEAT: Microwave, covered, until the desired temperature is reached or reheat in a frying pan or air fryer / instant pot, covered, on medium.

SERVE IT WITH: To make this a complete meal, it's best served with Mashed Cauliflower with Parmesan and Chives or Roasted Asparagus with Browned Butter.

PER SERVING

calories: 745 | fat: 52.7g | total carbs: 5.3g | fiber: 1.8g | protein: 64.1g

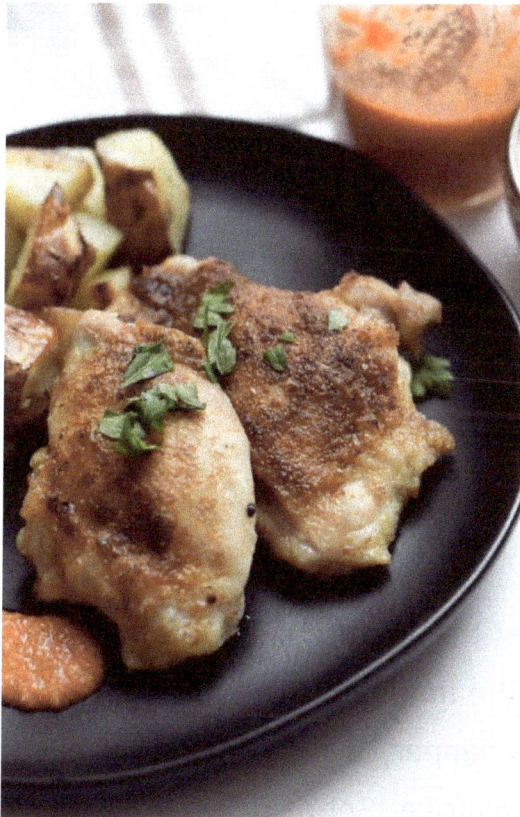

Lemon-Rosemary Roasted Cornish Hens
Macros: Fat 66% | Protein 30% | Carbs 4%

Prep time: 10 minutes | Cook time: 55 minutes | Serves 4

If you are only ever going to really master a single recipe, let it be this one! It's really simple. If you can cook chicken, you can cook cornish game hen.

This Cornish Game Hen Recipe is perfect for any occasion! The bright flavors of the lemon and rosemary will have everyone on the planet go crazy for having it and still wanting more.

4 Cornish game hen

Salt and freshly ground black pepper, to taste

3 tablespoons olive oil

4 sprigs fresh rosemary, plus 4 more sprigs for garnish

2 teaspoons paprika

1 lemon, quartered

24 cloves garlic

⅓ cup low-sodium chicken broth

⅓ cup dry white wine

1. Preheat the oven to 450°F (235°C).
2. Make the marinade: In a small bowl, stir together the salt, pepper, 2 tablespoons of olive oil, rosemary, and paprika. Set aside.

3. Clean and dry each hen. Squeeze the lemon juice inside the cavity and on the surface of each hen. Place 1 sprig of rosemary and 1 lemon wedge inside each hen. Evenly rub each hen with the marinade until well coated.

4. Place hens in a large roasting dish (at least an inch apart) and arrange garlic cloves around hens. (A bit of space between each hen leads to even browning and crispy skin.)

5. Place the roasting dish in the preheated oven and roast for about 25 minutes.

6. Reduce the oven temperature to 350°F (180°C).

7. Combine the remaining olive oil, chicken broth, and wine in a mixing bowl. Pour the mixture over hens and continue roasting for 25 minutes, or until hens are a deep golden color and reach at least 165°F (74°C) on a meat thermometer.

8. Remove the hens from the oven to a plate. Pour any remaining juices and garlic cloves to a medium saucepan. Cover the hens with aluminum foil to keep warm.

9. Boil the left juices and garlic cloves in the saucepan for 6 minutes until the liquid thickens to a sauce consistency.

10. Cut each hen half lengthwise into slices and place on serving plates. Pour the sauce and garlic cloves over them. Garnish with rosemary sprigs on top before serving.

STORAGE: Store in an airtight container in the fridge for up to 4 days or in the freezer for up to 1 month.

REHEAT: Microwave, covered, until the desired temperature is reached or reheat in a frying pan or air fryer / instant pot, covered, on medium.

SERVE IT WITH: To make this a complete meal, serve these hens alongside some mushrooms cooked in the hen juices.

PER SERVING

calories: 796 | fat: 58.3g | total carbs: 10.5g | fiber: 2.5g | protein: 59.8g

Grilled Tandori Boneless Chicken Thighs

Macros: Fat 68% | Protein 30% | Carbs 2%

Prep time:15 minutes | Cook time: 30 to 45 minutes | Serves 16

The flood of fat in chicken thighs is coming for you. We coat the thighs with great flavor of tandoori and the grilling will keep the thighs juicy. Without the bone, you can enjoy the chicken thighs entirely free.

2 (6-ounce / 170-g) containers plain Greek yogurt

2 tablespoons freshly grated ginger

½ teaspoon ground cloves

2 teaspoons kosher salt

1 teaspoon black pepper

4 teaspoons paprika

3 cloves garlic, minced

2 teaspoons ground cinnamon

2 teaspoons ground cumin

2 teaspoons ground coriander

16 chicken thighs

1 tablespoon olive oil

1. Mix together the yogurt, ginger, cloves, salt and pepper in a medium bowl. Add the paprika, garlic, cinnamon, cumin, and coriander. Stir well and set the marinade aside.

2. Rinse and pat dry the chicken thighs. Cut 4 to 5 slits in each thigh, then place in a plastic zip-top bag.

3. Pour the marinade over chicken, seal the bag and shake until it is coated completely. (Don't forget to press air out of it.). Put the bag in the refrigerator to marinate about 8 hours or overnight for the best results.

4. Preheat a grill to medium heat and lightly grease the grill grate with olive oil.

5. Get chicken out of the bag, and discard the marinade. Rub out the excess marinade with towel papers. Spray the chicken thighs with olive oil spray.

6. Grill the thighs about 2 minutes per side until nicely caramelized, then cook approximately 35 to 40 minutes until the internal temperature reaches at least 165°F (74°C) on an instant-read thermometer.

STORAGE: Store in an airtight container in the fridge for up to 4 days or in the freezer for up to 1 month.

REHEAT: Microwave, covered, until the desired temperature is reached or reheat in a frying pan or air fryer / instant pot, covered, on medium.

SERVE IT WITH: To make this a complete meal, it's best served with a whipped cucumber raita with plain Greek yogurt, crushed garlic, and a dash of salt.

PER SERVING

calories: 445 | fat: 33.8g | total carbs: 2.7g | fiber: 0.5g | protein: 32.9g

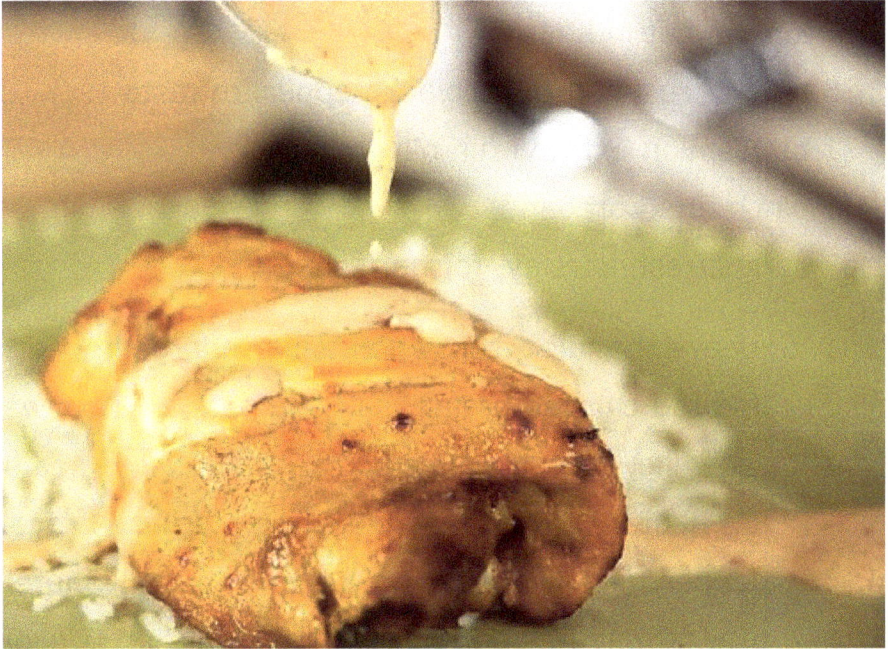

Lemon Herb Chicken Breasts
Macros: Fat 35% | Protein 63% | Carbs 2%

Prep time:10 minutes | Cook time: 25 to 30 minutes | Serves 2

If you're looking for an easy, simple, and drop-dead-delicious way to cook chicken breasts quickly, you've found it! It's guaranteed to win the hearts of friends and family!

2 skinless, boneless chicken breast halves

1 lemon, cut in half

Salt and freshly ground black pepper, to taste

1 tablespoon extra virgin olive oil

1 pinch dried oregano

2 sprigs fresh parsley, for garnish

1. Squeeze the juice from ½ lemon to a large bowl, then add the chicken breast, salt and pepper. Toss well.
2. Meanwhile, heat the olive oil in a skillet over medium-low heat. Add the seasoned chicken breast, oregano, pepper, and juice from remaining lemon. Sauté for 6 to 10 minutes per side until the chicken is cooked through.
3. Remove from the heat and garnish with fresh parsley.

STORAGE: Fried chicken left in the refrigerator is good only for 3 to 4 days.

REHEAT: To reheat, let it in the room temperature for an hour then place the chicken in an oven-safe dish, pour a cup of chicken broth in the bottom of the dish, and cover everything with foil. Place it in the oven, at 350ºF (180ºC), for about 25 minutes.

You can also set it on a plate covered and microwave it on medium for 2 to 5 minutes.

PER SERVING

calories: 337 | fat: 13.0g | total carbs: 2.0g | fiber: 0.3g | protein: 53.3g

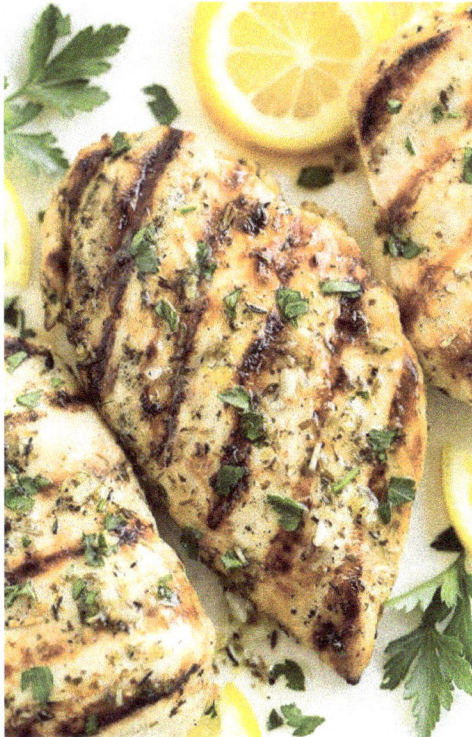

Lime Chicken Ginger
Macros: Fat 28% | Protein 66% | Carbs 6%

Prep time: 10 minutes | Cook time: 20 minutes | Serves 4

Chicken, a perfect meat to cook for any occasion. It's incredibly versatile and takes on flavors really well! Ginger and lime in the marinade used to produce this recipe create the ideal combination of flavors. The marinade can be made forwards and is easy to toss along with lime juice, lime zest, ginger, garlic, oil, sesame, and coriander.

And this lime chicken ginger is one meal that's perfect to make all year around. It is perfect to throw on the barbecue in the summer but is equally as good to grill in a pan and make a fresh salad or fajitas with any time of the year.

1½ pounds (680 g) boneless, skinless chicken breasts

¼ cup coconut aminos

2 tablespoons lime juice

2 teaspoons olive oil

1 teaspoon lime zest

1 teaspoon fresh ginger

Pinch red pepper flakes, to taste

1 teaspoon sesame seeds, toasted

1 tablespoon fresh cilantro, chopped

1. Put the breasts of chicken in a huge, shallow dish. Poke holes in the chicken using a fork. This helps the chicken to drink the marinade.
2. Fill a small bowl with the aminos coconut, lime juice, olive oil, lime zest, ginger and red pepper flakes and blend to combine. Pour the mixture over the chicken and allow to marinate in the fridge for at least 3 hours.
3. Place over medium to high heat on a large grill pan. Once the pan is hot, add the chicken to the grill pan and pour the extra marinade over the top. Cook, turning halfway through until the chicken become golden brown and caramelized outside, and cooked for about 10 to 15 minutes all the way through.
4. Before eating, sprinkle with the red pepper flakes, sesame seeds and coriander.

STORAGE: Keeping foods separate and well covered helps to combat potential cross-contamination. store it in a plastic container in the fridge for up to 3 to 4 days or in the freezer for up to 3 weeks

REHEAT: Microwave, grill, covered, or reheated in frying pan or air fryer / instant pot. Don't reheat leftovers more than once. This is because the more times you cool and reheat food, the higher the risk of food poisoning.

SERVE IT WITH: Serve with salad or steamed low-carb vegetables.

PER SERVING

calories: 232 | fat: 7.2g | total carbs: 3.8g | fiber: 0.2g | protein: 38.5g

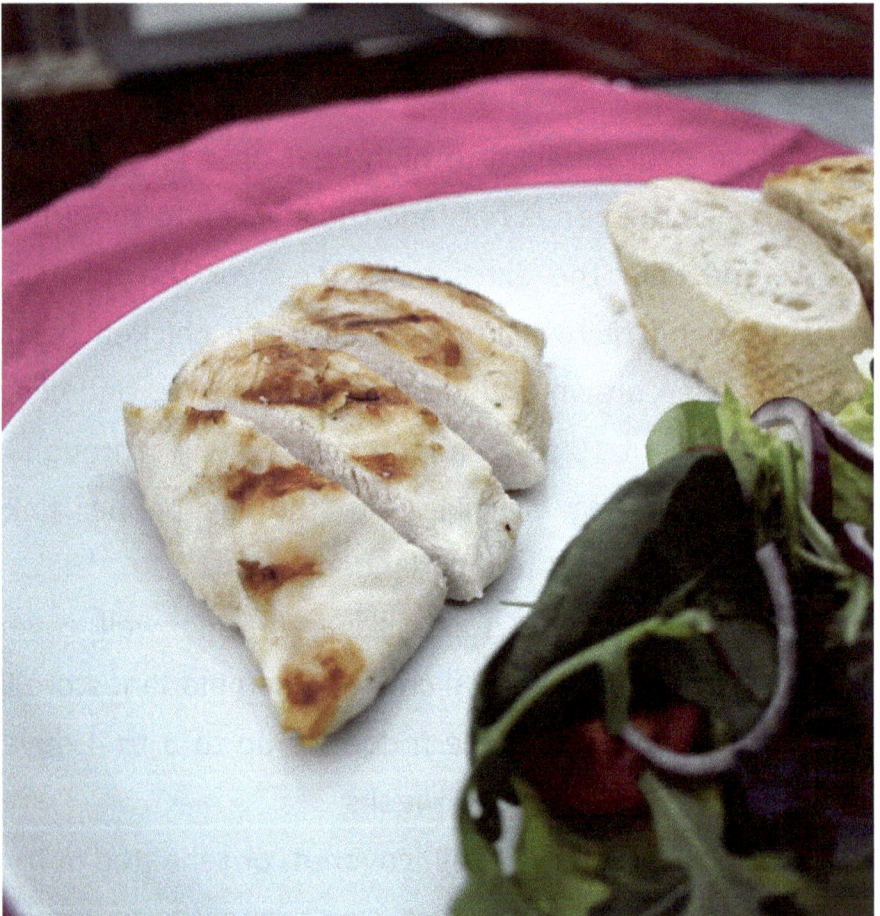

Roast Chicken with Broccoli And Garlic
Macros: Fat 68% | Protein 23% | Carbs 9%

Prep time: 10 minutes | Cook time: 45 minutes | Serves 4

Roast Chicken with broccoli and garlic -yum! It's a quick, savory, nutritious, cheap keto meal. Works well as a short dinner, or a balanced lunch box. It'll become a favorite go-to. Cooked chicken and broccoli in 45 minutes in a garlic butter sauce, all in one oven!

CHICKEN LEGS:

4 (5-ounce / 140-g) chicken legs

1 teaspoon garlic powder

2 tablespoons olive oil

1 tablespoon Italian seasoning

½ teaspoon salt (if not have salt in the Italian seasoning)

Freshly ground black pepper, to taste

GARLIC BUTTER:

4 tablespoons unsalted butter, softened

2 garlic cloves, pressed

1 tablespoon fresh parsley, finely chopped

Salt and freshly ground black pepper, to taste

BROCCOLI:

20 ounces (567 g) broccoli

Salt, to taste

1. Preheat oven to 400°F (205°C).
2. Season both sides of chicken legs with salt, garlic powder, black pepper, and Italian seasoning.
3. Heat 1 tablespoon olive oil in a large skillet or cast iron pan over medium-high heat. Cook chicken breasts 4 to 5 minutes per side or until browned and cooked through and reaches 165°F (74°C).
4. Cut the broccoli into florets when the chicken is in the skillet, and slice the stem. In a saucepan, boil in light salted water for 5 minutes. Drain and put the water on the lid to keep it warm.
5. In a bowl, mix all the ingredients for the garlic butter. And serve with chicken legs and broccoli.

STORAGE: store it in a glass or plastic container in the fridge for up to 3 to 4 days or in the freezer for up to 3 weeks.

REHEAT: Microwave, grill, covered, or reheated in frying pan or air fryer / instant pot. Don't reheat leftovers more than once.

SERVE IT WITH: Serve with broccoli and garlic butter on the chicken.

PER SERVING

calories: 494 | fat: 37.6g | total carbs: 12.1g | fiber: 4.1g | protein: 28.0g

Mushrooms And Chicken with Tomato Cream

Macros: Fat 69% | Protein 24% | Carbs 7%

Prep time: 10 minutes | Cook time: 1 hour 30 minutes | Serves 4

This mushrooms and chicken with tomato cream is full of flavor and ready in less than 90 minutes. Elegant enough for a date night, fast enough and easy enough for a week-end dinner. It's sure to be a family favorite! I love this Chicken with Mushroom and Tomato cream! It's just so delicious. It is super-fast and simple

7 ounces (198 g) skinless, boneless chicken breasts

1 tablespoon olive oil

Ground black pepper and sea salt, to taste

2 tablespoons salted butter

3 garlic cloves, minced

6 cremini mushrooms, thinly sliced

1 cup heavy whipping cream

3 ounces (85 g) Parmesan cheese, finely grated

4 ounces (113 g) fresh tomatoes, diced

Fresh basil, for garnish

1. Season the chicken breasts generously with salt and pepper on both sides.

2. Heat up the olive oil over medium to high heat in a large skillet. Pan-sear the chicken breasts until each side is golden brown and caramelized, about 4 to 5 minutes. Take off the pan and cover to keep warm.
3. Add the butter, garlic and mushrooms to the same pan, reduce the heat to medium-low, and sauté until the garlic is fragrant and the mushrooms have released their liquid.
4. In the pan add the heavy cream, Parmesan and diced tomatoes. To thicken, mix in and let simmer, about 10 minutes.
5. Add the chicken back to the saucepan and cook until completely cooked. Taste, and if necessary, add more salt and pepper.
6. Plate and top with fresh basil.

STORAGE: store it in a glass or plastic container in the fridge for up to 3 days or in the freezer for up to 2 weeks.

REHEAT: Microwave, grill, covered, or reheated in frying pan or air fryer / instant pot.

SERVE IT WITH: Serve with Loaded Cauliflower Salad.

PER SERVING

calories: 326 | fat: 25.6g | total carbs: 5.8g | fiber: 0.4g | protein: 18.5g

Simple Chicken Tonnato

Macros: Fat 71% | Protein 28% | Carbs 1%

Prep time: 10 minutes | Cook time: 20 minutes | Serves 4

Get your keto on with this amazing and simple chicken tonnato keto dish! Fall in love with fresh basil and rich tuna and enveloping savory chicken. It doesn't get much more keto-taste than this!

TONNATO SAUCE:

4 ounces (113 g) tuna

2 garlic cloves

¼ cup fresh basil, chopped

1 teaspoon dried parsley

2 tablespoons lemon juice

½ cup mayonnaise, keto-friendly

¼ cup olive oil

½ teaspoon salt

¼ teaspoon ground black pepper

CHICKEN:

1½ pounds (680g) chicken breasts

Salt, to taste

Water, as needed

7 ounces (198 g) leafy green

1. Mix all of the sauce ingredients in an immersion blender or in a food processor. Reserve the Tonnato sauce to allow the aromas to grow.
2. In a pot, put the chicken breasts with only enough lightly salted water to cover them. Bring to a boil.
3. Let simmer for around 15 minutes over medium heat, or until the chicken is completely cooked through. When you are using a meat thermometer, when finished, it will say 16 5°F (7 4°C).
4. Enable the breasts of chicken to rest, at least 10 minutes before slicing.
5. Place the leafy greens on the serving plates, and top with the sliced chicken. Pour the sauce over the chicken and serve with a slice of fresh lemon and extra capers.

STORAGE: store it in a glass or plastic container in the fridge for up to 3 to 4 days or in the freezer for up to 1 month.

REHEAT: Grill, skillet, or reheated in frying pan or air fryer / instant pot.

SERVE IT WITH: Serve with beef stock and cauliflower rice.

PER SERVING

calories: 652 | fat: 51.3g | total carbs: 2.8g | fiber: 0.8g | protein: 43.2g

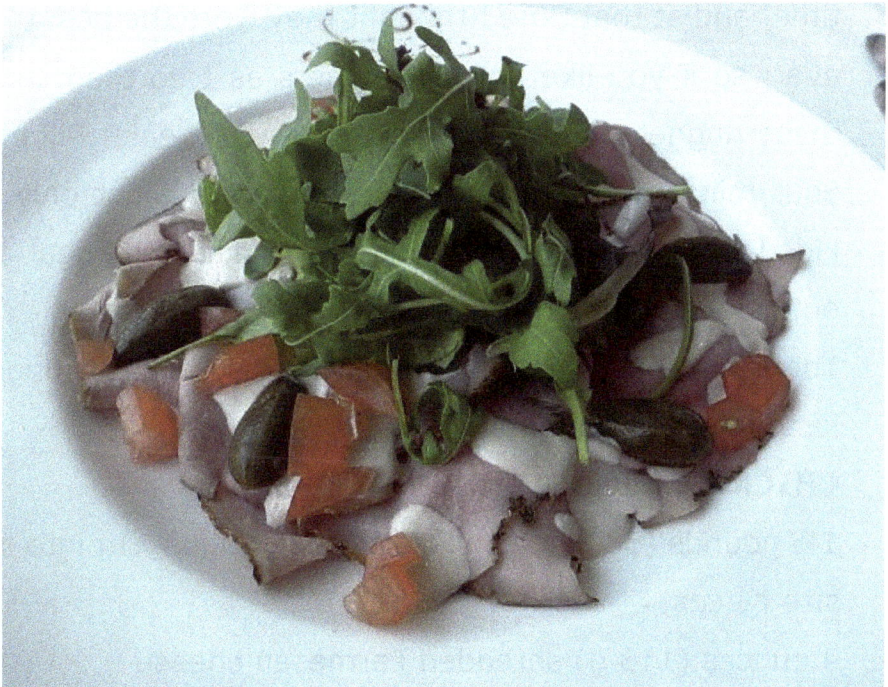

Chicken Nuggets with Fried Green Bean and Bbq-Mayo

Marcos: Fat 71% | Protein 24% | Carbs 5%

Prep time: 20 minutes | Cook time:25 minutes | Serves 6

Looking for another yummy scrummy keto meal? The Chicken nuggets with fried green bean is what you are looking for. As a young boy I used to eat nuggets all the time, and at that time I thought they were the best thing ever, so if you like normal nuggets as I do then surely these nuggets with BBQ-mayo and fried beans will blow your mind my friend. Chicken nuggets are not only for kids to enjoy, so make yourself this delicious meal and enjoy it regardless of your age.

There is no problem if you want to use chicken fingers instead of the nuggets.

CHICKEN NUGGETS:

1½ pounds (680 g) boneless chicken thighs, cut into bite size pieces

4 ounces (113 g) shredded Parmesan cheese

1 tablespoon onion powder

¼ tablespoon salt

¼ tablespoon ground black pepper

1 egg

1 tablespoon coconut oil

GREEN BEAN FRIES:

8 ounces (227 g) fresh green beans, trimmed

1 tablespoon coconut oil

¾ cup mayonnaise, keto-friendly

½ tablespoon smoked chili powder

1 tablespoon garlic powder

Salt and freshly ground black pepper, to taste

1. Put the Parmesan, onion powder, salt and pepper in a medium bowl and stir them till they are mixed very well

2. In another bowl, add the egg and whisk until it gets frothy.

3. Start Dipping the chicken pieces in the egg, and make sure to cover them entirely.

4. Coat the chicken nuggets in the Parmesan mixture by dipping them and shake off any excess.

5. Melt the coconut oil in a large skillet over medium heat, then fry the chicken nuggets on each side for 5 minutes until they become golden brown and cooked through.

6. Heat up coconut oil in a large skillet to medium-high, then put the trimmed beans and fry them for a

couple of minutes. They should be crispy. Season the beans with salt before serving.

7. Now for the BBQ-mayo sauce, you should prepare a medium bowl and mix the mayonnaise, smoked chili powder, garlic powder, and a little bit of salt and pepper together, then stir very well and refrigerate for 30 minutes before serving.

STORAGE: Nuggets unfortunately last only for a day or two in the refrigerator. To maximize the quality of the nuggets. Wrap them with aluminum foil, or put them in a shallow airtight container.

REHEAT: It heats well in the microwave, but if you wanted them to be a bit tough then place the nuggets on a parchment paper lined cookie sheet, and make sure you preheat the oven to 35 0 °F (180°C) , keeping them in there for 10 minutes will be enough to get them tasty and crunchy again.

SERVE IT WITH: There are a lot of things that could go along with this dish. Such as broccoli rice. The choices are not limited to certain things.

PER SERVING

calories: 644 | fat: 51.0g | total carbs: 8.5g | fiber: 1.7g | protein: 37.7g

Keto Fried Chicken with Broccoli

Marcos: Fat 85% | Protein 12% | Carbs 3%

Prep time: 5 minutes | Cook time: 15 minutes | Serves 3

Not many things could be done in 20 minutes, right? Well, you might want to reconsider that opinion because this luscious dish of broccoli and fried chicken takes only 20 minutes to prepare. I remember the first time I made this dish. It tastes like something that I would order from a Chinese restaurant but even better. It saves me through many days when I was busy, and it's delicious at the same time, so what are you waiting for? Prepare the ingredients and get yourself ready for an enjoyable journey.

9 ounces (255 g) broccoli

3½ ounces (99 g) butter

10 ounces (284 g) boneless chicken thighs

Salt and freshly ground black pepper, to taste

½ cup keto-friendly mayonnaise

1. Wash and cut the broccoli and the stem into small pieces.
2. Heat up a good amount of butter in a big frying pan where you will be able to fit both the broccoli and the chicken.

3. Season the chicken with salt and pepper, then fry over medium heat for 5 minutes on each side, or until it turns golden brown and cooked through. You can check by using a cooking thermometer in the thickest part, it gets fully cooked when it reaches 180°F (82°C)
4. Add a bit more butter and place the broccoli in the frying pan, and fry for another 2 minutes.
5. Season to taste with salt and pepper, and pour the remained butter on top, then serve.

STORAGE: place the leftovers in an air tight container and put it in the fridge. It lasts up to 3 days in the fridge. It lasts for about 1 month in the freezer in a freezer-safe container.

REHEAT: You could reheat it in the microwave with no problem, or in the oven at 35 0 °F (18 0 ℃) for 15 minutes.

SERVE IT WITH: You could serve it with a keto salad of your choice such as the grilled vegetable salad with pesto.

PER SERVING

calories: 653 | fat: 61.7g | total carbs: 6.2g | fiber: 2.3g | protein: 19.5g

Roasted Chicken Thighs and Cauliflower Puree

Marcos: Fat 70% | Protein 25% | Carbs 4%

Prep time: 3 hours 15 minutes | Cook time: 35 minutes | Serves 6

Since I'm attempting to constrain the number of carbs, I eat around evening time, I got a couple of cauliflower heads and transformed them into the smoothest, the richest purée which was the ideal backup to the succulent, flavorful chicken. What's more, the garlic! Gracious, the garlic. You folks, I could most likely live off broiled garlic. I made them alongside the chicken. At the point when cooked, the garlic turns out to be sweet and subtle, and draining them out of their papery skins is genuinely the best time you can have with your pants on.

CHICKEN THIGHS:

3 pounds (1.4 kg) chicken thighs, 2 thighs per serving, skin on and bone in

4 tablespoons olive oil

4 tablespoons lemon juice

2 tablespoons red wine vinegar

3 tablespoons finely cut fresh oregano.

2 tablespoons finely cut fresh thyme

2 garlic diced cloves

2 teaspoons salt

1 teaspoon black pepper

CAULIFLOWER PUREE:

1 pound (454 g) cauliflower, cut into florets

3 ounces (85 g) Parmesan cheese, grated

3 tablespoons melted butter, unsalted

½ lemon, zest and juice

1 tablespoon olive oil

CHICKEN THIGHS:

1. Put the olive oil, lemon juice, red wine vinegar, oregano, thyme, diced garlic cloves, salt, and pepper in bowl or a large zip lock bag, then add the thighs and flip it on sides in the mixture to fully coat.

2. Seal or cover, and put in the fridge for 3 hours. Keep turning them every now and then for a better taste.

3. Heat the oven in advance to 400°F (205°C). Place one large baking tray, or two regular ones with parchment paper.

4. Take out the chicken thighs from the mixture, and gently put them skin-side up, on top of the tray(s).

5. Keep them in the oven for about 30 to 35 minutes, or use a cooking thermometer, and make sure that the internal temperature is 165°F (74°C), and that the skin color is golden brown. After that let it rest for

10 minutes before you serve it with the cauliflower mash.

CAULIFLOWER MASH:

1. Boil a pot of slightly salted on high heat, then add on the cauliflower to the pot and boil for 2 to 5 minutes, or until tender but remain firm. Strain all the cauliflower florets in a colander, and get rid of the water.

2. Put the cauliflower in a food processor, along with the cheese, butter, lemon zest and juice, and olive oil. Keep pulsing until they gain a creamy and smooth consistency. You have the choice of using an immersion blender.

3. Salt and pepper to taste . You could put more butter or olive oil if you wish.

STORAGE: The purée could be prepared in advance and kept in the refrigerator for up to 3 days. It lasts for a month in the freezer, but make sure to keep it in a freezer-safe container. The chicken will remain for 3 to 4 days in the refrigerator in an airtight container.

REHEAT: In order to warm it up, you can place it on a dry skillet over medium heat until it gets warm enough.

SERVE IT WITH: It can be served with any keto salad of your choice. I recommend the classic Greek salad for a kind of variation.

PER SERVING

calories: 725 | fat: 57.1g | total carbs: 9.1g | fiber: 2.4g | protein: 43.5g

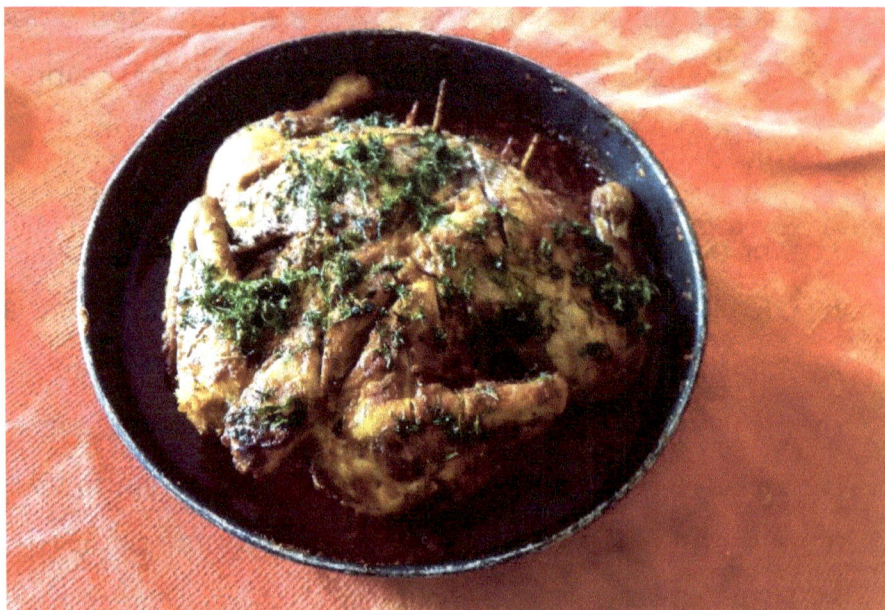

Delicious Fried Chicken with Broccoli
Marcos: Fat 72% | Protein 22% | Carbs 6%

Prep time: 10 minutes | Cook time: 25 minutes | Serves 4

There are too many recipes that could be done with chicken thighs, and for that every time I try a new one. Sometimes they are yummy sometimes not, so let me say this clearly. This fried thigh with broccoli and butter is one of the best recipes that I have discovered. If you are looking for a simple, basic, and flavorful approach to cook chicken. You have discovered it! These chicken thighs with broccoli and butter have become a regular in my household since they are so exquisite.

5 ounces (142 g) separated butter

1½ pounds (680 g) chicken thighs, boneless

Salt and freshly ground black pepper, to taste

1 pound (454 g) broccoli

½ leek

1 tablespoon garlic, powder

1. Put half of the butter over medium high heat in a large frying pan to melt it.
2. Add salt and pepper to the chicken for seasoning, and then place it on pan. Keep flipping the chicken for 20 to 25 minutes (depends on the thighs size) until it

turns brown on both of the sides, then remove them it from the pan, but keep it warm by covering it with aluminum foil or in the oven on over low heat.

3. While the thighs are in the oven, wash the broccoli including the stem and trim it. Slice it into small pieces. Rinse and wash the leek, but be careful to remove any sandy deposits between the layers. chop the leek into big pieces.

4. In a different skillet, melt the rest of the butter on medium heat, then add in the salt and pepper, and the garlic powder. Put the leek to them, and start stirring slowly until it starts to get softer, then put the broccoli. Cook it for about 5 minutes, until it becomes tender.

5. Serve the vegetables and chicken with an extra amount melted butter on top.

STORAGE: The chicken thighs could be stored in the refrigerator and will last for up to 4 days in the, and for 2 months in the freezer, but make sure you keep it in freezer-safe container.

REHEAT: It heats perfectly in the microwave, but you can also heat it in the oven. Heat your oven in advance to 350ºF (180ºC). Place the chicken wings on a baking sheet in a single layer. Put the wings in the preheated oven for about 15 to 20 minutes .

SERVE IT WITH: It could be served with keto salads of your choice such as the classic Greek salad .

PER SERVING

calories: 602 | fat: 48.3g | total carbs: 10.3g | fiber: 3.2g | protein: 32.8g

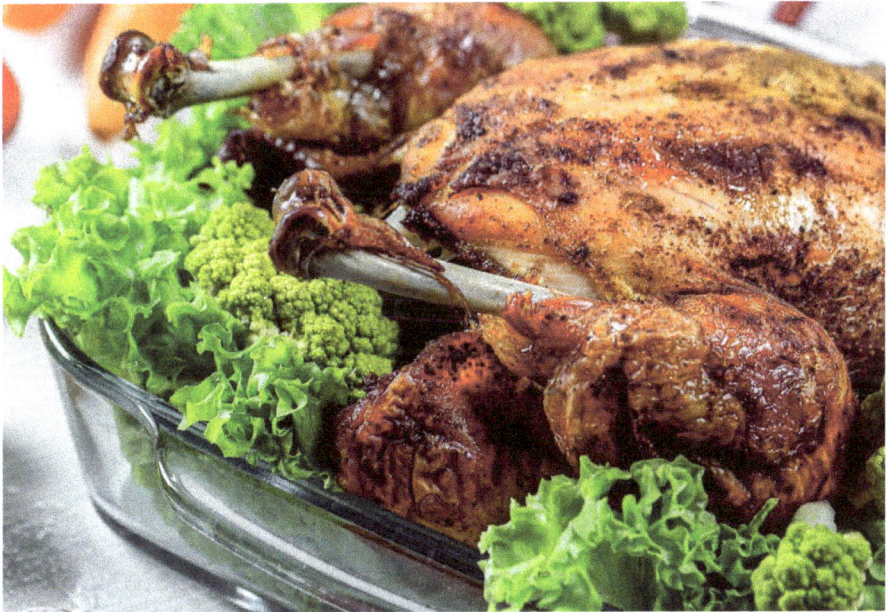

Rotisserie Chicken and Keto Chili-Flavored Béarnaise Sauce

Marcos: Fat 69% | Protein 30% | Carbs 1%

Prep time: 10 minutes | Cook time: 15 minutes | Serves 6

To Rotisserie or not to Rotisserie, that is the question! Well, it's definitely one of the most delicious dishes to me. I have tried Rotisserie chicken in many places, but it never tastes as good as the homemade one. I realized that I don't need a cook to make me Rotisserie chicken because the world's best Rotisserie chicken could come out of your own kitchen. What do you need in order to make that happen? All you need is chicken, few spices, an oven, and love.

2 rotisserie chickens

4 egg yolks

2 tablespoons white wine vinegar

½ tablespoon onion powder

1 finely chopped and deseeded red chili pepper

10 ounces (284 g) butter

Salt and freshly ground black pepper, to taste

3 ounces (85 g) leafy vegetables

1. Split the chicken into two pieces, and make a fresh leafy salad or basically another side dish of your choice.

2. Crack the eggs and take only egg yolks, then put them into a heat-resistant bowl. Mix the wine vinegar, chili and onion powder in a mug, then put the butter in a saucepan and melt it.

3. Slowly beat the egg yolks and add the butter one drop at a time into the yolk while whisking. Increase the pace as the sauce thickens. Continue to whisk until you are done with all the butter. You'll see that white milk protein has accumulated at the pan's bottom; however, it should be removed.

4. Put the vinegar in, then stir together with salt and pepper to add taste. Make sure to keep the sauce warm.

5. Serve it with green salad and a fried chicken or any other side dish of your choice, personally I prefer the green sal ad because it adds variation to the taste.

STORAGE: It lasts for up to 4 days in the refrigerator, and for 2 months in the freezer, but make sure you keep it in freezer-safe container.

REHEAT: To heat Rotisserie chicken you'll need to place it in an oven-safe dish, and roast in the oven for 25 minutes at 350ºF (180ºC).

SERVE IT WITH: You can serve it with any kind of green salad, two of my favorites are caprese zoodles and classic Greek salad.

PER SERVING

calories: 505 | fat: 38.9g | total carbs: 2.1g | fiber: 0.4g | protein: 37.5g

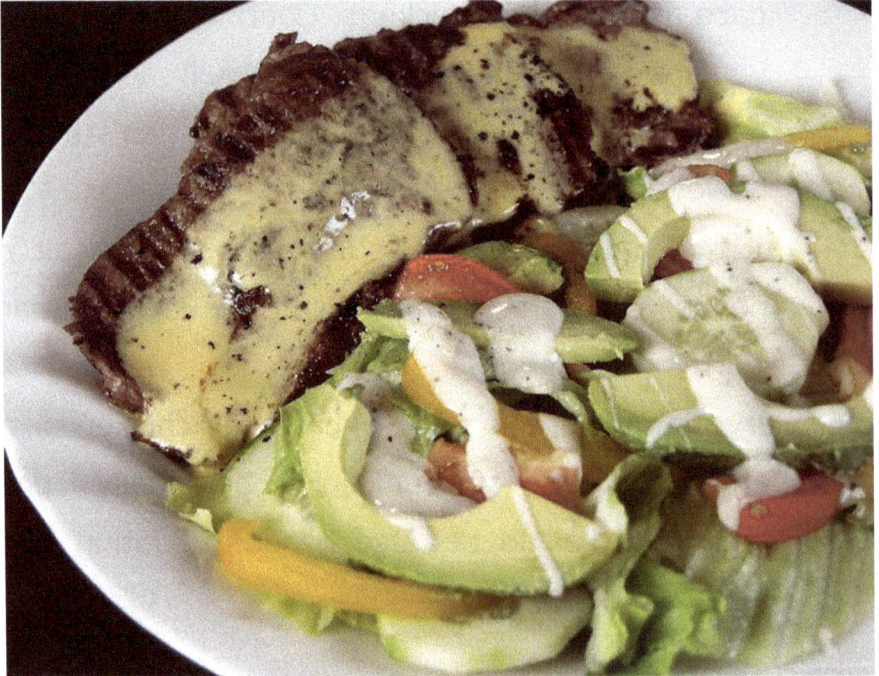

Chicken Wings and Blue Cheese Dip
Macros: Fat 58% | Protein 39%| Carbs 3%

Prep time: 1 hour | Cook time: 25 minutes | Serves 4

Something I learned in my early ages is that you simply cannot enjoy chicken wings without the blue cheese dressing. To me it feels like a rule that should be taught in school, and the equation should be that chicken wings plus blue cheese dip equals happiness. If you have never tried the blue cheese dip with chicken wings then what are you waiting for? Let your tongue enjoy the creaminess of the cheese with the mouth-watering wings.

You could have any other dip of your choice such as the curry sauce or the traditional hot sauce.

⅓ cup mayonnaise, keto-friendly

¼ cup sour cream

3 tablespoons lemon juice

¼ tablespoon garlic powder

¼ tablespoon salt

¼ cup heavy whipping cream

3 ounces (85 g) blue cheese, crumbled

2 pounds (907 g) chicken wings

2 tablespoons olive oil

¼ tablespoon garlic powder

1 garlic clove, minced

1 teaspoon salt

¼ tablespoon ground black pepper

2 ounces (57 g) Parmesan cheese, grated

1. Put the mayonnaise, sour cream, lemon juice, garlic powder, salt, and cream in a large bowl, and whisk to combine. Add the blue cheese crumbles in and mix well.

2. Let it chill for about 45 minutes before you serve it. You can use this dressing over salads or as I recommend as a dip for the wings or vegetables.

3. Prepare the chicken wings: place the wings in large bowl. Add the olive oil, garlic powder, minced garlic, salt, and black pepper. Start stirring slowly in order to coat the chicken. Let it marinate in the fridge for 30 minutes.

4. Preheat the oven to 425ºF (220ºC).

5. Grill or bake in the preheated oven for about 25 minutes, or until brown and tender; the skin should be crispy.

6. Carefully take out the wings and place them in a large bowl, then add the Parmesan cheese. Finally, put the

wings in the cheese until they are coated, and Serve warm.

REHEAT: Preheat your oven to 350 ºF (180 ºC). Place the chicken wings on a baking sheet in a single layer. Put the wings in the preheated oven for about 15 to 20 minutes.

STORAGE: The chicken wings could last for four days in the refrigerator, and make sure that you wrap the cheese dip in parchment or wax paper and keep it in the refrigerator because otherwise it won't last for more than 2 days.

SERVE IT WITH: You could add your own choice of vegetables to go along with the wings. Or you can serve it with sliced cucumber or celery.

PER SERVING

calories: 658 | fat: 42.8g | total carbs: 6.0g | fiber: 0.3g | protein: 59.6g

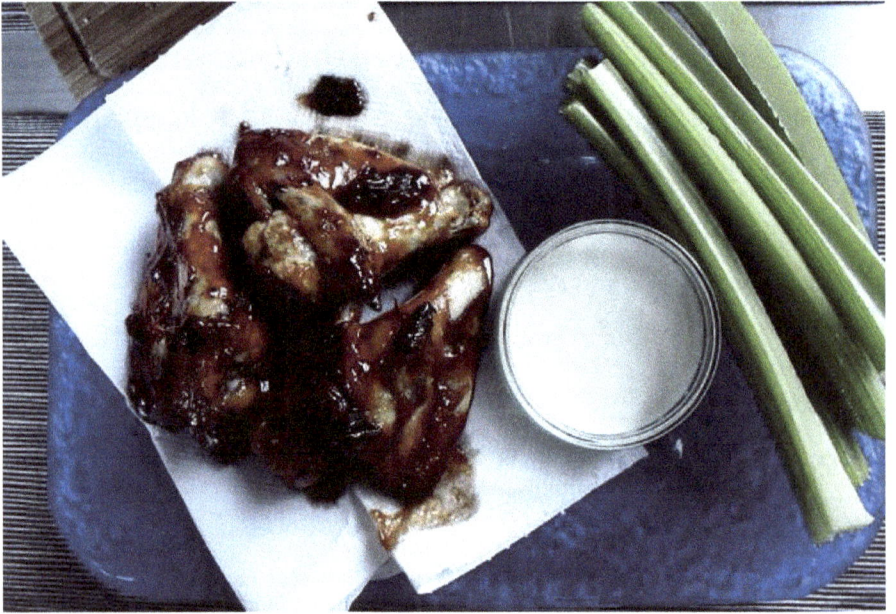

www.ingramcontent.com/pod-product-compliance
Lightning Source LLC
Chambersburg PA
CBHW050753030426
42336CB00012B/1804